Disaster Me

Editor

MARY SHOWSTARK

PHYSICIAN ASSISTANT CLINICS

www.physicianassistant.theclinics.com

Consulting Editor
JAMES A. VAN RHEE

October 2019 • Volume 4 • Number 4

ELSEVIER

1600 John F. Kennedy Boulevard • Suite 1800 • Philadelphia, Pennsylvania, 19103-2899

http://www.theclinics.com

PHYSICIAN ASSISTANT CLINICS Volume 4, Number 4
October 2019 ISSN 2405-7991, ISBN-13: 978-0-323-68191-9

Editor: Jessica McCool
Developmental Editor: Casey Potter

Physician Assistant Clinics (ISSN: 2405–7991) is published quarterly by Elsevier Inc., 360 Park Avenue South, New York, NY 10010-1710. Months of issue are January, April, July, and October. Periodicals postage paid at New York, NY and additional mailing offices. Subscription prices are $150.00 per year (US individuals), $205.00 (US institutions), $100.00 (US students), $150.00 (Canadian individuals), $257.00 (Canadian institutions), $100.00 (Canadian students), $150.00 (international individuals), $257.00 (international institutions), and $100.00 (international students). Foreign air speed delivery is included in all *Clinics* subscription prices. All prices are subject to change without notice. POSTMASTER: Send address changes to *Physician Assistant Clinics*, Elsevier Periodicals Customer Service, 11830 Westline Industrial Drive, St. Louis, MO 63146. Customer Service Health Sciences Division, Subscription Customer Service, 3251 Riverport Lane, Maryland Heights, MO 63043. **Customer Service: 1-800-654-2452 (U.S. and Canada); 314-447-8871 (outside U.S. and Canada). Fax: 314-447-8029. E-mail: journalscustomerservice-usa@elsevier.com (for print support); journalsonlinesupport-usa@elsevier.com (for online support).**

Reprints. For copies of 100 or more, of articles in this publication, please contact the Commercial Reprints Department, Elsevier Inc., 360 Park Avenue South, New York, NY 10010-1710. Tel. 212-633-3874; Fax: 212-633-3820; E-mail: reprints@elsevier.com.

Physician Assistant Clinics is covered in *EMBASE/Excerpta Medica and ESCI.*

3. Complete the CME Test and Evaluation. Participants must achieve a score of 70% on the test. All CME Tests and Evaluations must be completed online.

CME INQUIRIES/SPECIAL NEEDS

For all CME inquiries or special needs, please contact elsevierCME@elsevier.com.

Contributors

CONSULTING EDITOR

JAMES A. VAN RHEE, MS, PA-C
Associate Professor, Program Director, Yale School of Medicine, Yale Physician Assistant Online Program, New Haven, Connecticut

EDITOR

MARY SHOWSTARK, MS, PA-C
Instructor, Yale School of Medicine, Physician Assistant Online Program, Yale University, New Haven, Connecticut

AUTHORS

JAMLA RIZEK BERGMAN, MSN, RN, CEN, CPEN, TCRN, NREMT-P
Clinical Coordinator, Detroit Medical Center Sinai Grace Hospital, Detroit, Michigan

BRANDON M. CARIUS, MPAS, PA-C
San Antonio Military Medical Center, JBSA Fort Sam Houston, San Antonio, Texas

AMELIA M. DURAN-STANTON, PhD, DSc, MPAS, PA-C
US Army, Fort Sam Houston, Texas

ANDREW D. FISHER, MPAS, PA-C
Medical Command, Texas Army National Guard, Austin, Texas; Texas A&M College of Medicine, Temple, Texas

GIACOMO FLORIO, PA-C
Physician's Assistant, St. James Hospital, Hornell, New York; Emergency Department, Highland Hospital, Rochester, New York

STEPHAN C. KESTERSON, MPAS, PA-C
Team Chief, Expeditionary Medical Decontamination Team, Omaha, Nebraska

BRYAN LOVEJOY, DNP, FNP-BC
Nurse Practitioner, Department of Medicine, Northwell Health, Disaster Medical Assistance Team NY4, Smithtown, New York

JAMES E. PATRICK, MS, PA-C
Aeromedical Physician Assistant, Medical Detachment, Florida Army National Guard, Starke, Florida; Physician Assistant, Department of Emergency Medicine, Oakes Medical Center, Oakes, North Dakota

JOSHUA K. RADI, PhD, PA-C
Physician Assistant, 93rd Weapons of Mass Destruction-Civil Support Team, Hawaii
Army National Guard, Kapolei, Hawaii; Physician Assistant, Department of Orthopaedic
Surgery, Tripler Army Medical Center, Clinical Educator, Department of Surgery,
University of Hawaii John A. Burns School of Medicine, Honolulu, Hawaii

LARRY REEDER, RRPT, BS Technology
Duke Energy Florida, Crystal River, Florida

MARY SHOWSTARK, MS, PA-C
Instructor, Yale School of Medicine, Physician Assistant Online Program, Yale University,
New Haven, Connecticut

RALPH R. STANTON Jr, MA
Graduate Certificate in Geographic Information Systems (GIS), U.S. Army Veteran
(Former Medical Service Corps Officer), San Antonio, Texas

NATHANIEL J. TAYLOR, MPAS, PA-C
Adjunct Professor of Physician Assistant Studies, Northern Arizona University, Medical
Director, 91st Weapons of Mass Destruction Team, Phoenix, Arizona

Contents

Mary Showstark and Bryan Lovejoy

This article defines crisis standards of care (CSC) and gives a brief overview of how it is used in a disaster setting. The article also briefly describes how triage works in a disaster setting, as well as how to work with limited supplies and staffing. The article also touches on the provider's role when using CSC and their liability in times of disaster.

Ralph R. Stanton Jr and Amelia M. Duran-Stanton

When people are displaced by disasters, medical professionals should consider residence, resilience, and resources interrelated with vulnerable populations. What is a vulnerable population and whom does it comprise? What is social vulnerability? Where are vulnerable populations located? Where do people reside when displaced by a disaster? What is resilience? Where are the resources for response and survival? Will thematic maps help visualize vulnerable populations over space and time? Although no panacea exists to reduce social vulnerability, spatial analysis of human landscapes helps visualize vulnerable populations as a whole, rather than the overall sum of the parts within a built environment.

Ralph R. Stanton Jr and Amelia M. Duran-Stanton

"Is less really more?" Medical professionals in clinic and hospital settings need to account for convergence behavior to disrupt responder communications in disaster, especially when there is a mass casualty situation that overwhelms local resources. Emergency management is an art linked to different types of improvisation. Incident commanders and other key stakeholders will require situation reports. Ultimately, there is no panacea to facilitate dialogue, but it may behoove an organization to design a communications strategy and viably use the IDEA Model to distribute key messages with PACE: (1) Primary, (2) Alternate, (3) Contingent, and (4) Emergent forms of communication.

Stephan C. Kesterson and Nathaniel J. Taylor

Chemical warfare agents are designed to injure, incapacitate, or kill their intended targets, classified by their physiochemical properties and physiologic effects to health. Industrial chemicals have the potential to be used for nefarious intent, although accidental release also poses significant risks to populations and local communities. Recognition of various chemical toxicants by clinicians may facilitate early diagnosis and medical management for exposed individuals.

This article discusses what radiation is and how people are exposed, both to naturally occurring as well as man-made radioactive material. It also discusses methods used to recognize the hazard, the effects on exposed individuals, how to handle contaminated patients, treatment options, as well as pathways to follow when responding to the incident as well as the patients.

Biological agents are a legitimate threat for state-level warfare and rogue actor terror. There are key clinical features of most of these conditions that indicate their likelihood with specific definitive diagnostics and treatments available for each. Although it is difficult to maintain a suspicion for these biological agents, multiple patients presenting at the same time with atypical symptoms should prompt early engagement of public health authorities. Modern advancements in engineering technology are revolutionizing the world creating the potential for both amazing and catastrophic outcomes in the biological world.

This article focuses primarily on terrorist vehicle attack, which has become a global threat. Awareness, preparation, medical response, and mitigation measures need to be implemented in order to adapt to this threat. The primary goal is prevention; however, reducing morbidity/mortality of these attacks is paramount if prevention fails. This article also discusses emerging vehicle-based threats that have become prevalent in most Western countries. Enhancing awareness for the probability of these vehicle attacks (explosive and ramming) provides first responders the ability to rehearse tactical/medical response procedures and improve the incident response effort based on the most likely scenario.

The article offers providers the background on blast devices, discusses previous explosive events, and explains how the provider can respond. Information is given on types of blasts, scene safety, and prehospital and hospital care of blast victims. Blast physics and the injuries commonly seen after the explosion are discussed.

Disaster Medicine

PHYSICIAN ASSISTANT CLINICS

SERIES OF RELATED INTEREST

Medical Clinics of North America
https://www.medical.theclinics.com/
Primary Care: Clinics in Office Practice
https://www.primarycare.theclinics.com/

THE CLINICS ARE AVAILABLE ONLINE!
Access your subscription at:
www.theclinics.com

Foreword

Disaster Medicine

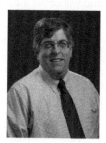

James A. Van Rhee, MS, PA-C
Consulting Editor

The American Academy of Physician Assistants (AAPA) has a policy related to the physician assistants (PAs) response in disaster situations. Below are two of the core guidelines from this policy.[1]

- AAPA believes PAs are established and valued participants in the health care system of this country and are fully qualified to deliver medical services during disaster relief efforts.
- AAPA supports educational activities that prepare the profession for participation in disaster medical planning, training, and response.

The first guideline states that PAs are qualified to deliver medical services during disaster relief efforts, and the second states that educational activities that prepare PAs to participate should be available to PAs. With that in mind, this issue provides an overview of disaster medicine and what a PA should know in some of these situations. This is not a comprehensive review; there are a number of other resources available if you would like more information.

In this issue, we provide information on some of the more focused topics in disaster medicine. Taylor and Kesterson provide a review of chemical threats; Taylor and Reeder discuss radioactive contamination. Showstark, the guest editor for this issue, discusses treating patients after bombs and blasts; Radi and Patrick discuss the care associated with vehicle blasts. Taylor and Kesterson also review high-risk pathogens. Fisher and Carius discuss stopping the bleed in a disaster. Not every article in this issue has to do with the care of patients. The care of the responders to disasters is discussed by Florio and Bergman; Lovejoy and Showstark describe the standard of care in crisis, and Duran-Stanton and Stanton discuss the importance of responder communication in a disaster and discuss the residence, resilience, and resources in vulnerable populations in a disaster.

Physician Assist Clin 4 (2019) xi–xii
https://doi.org/10.1016/j.cpha.2019.07.001
2405-7991/19/© 2019 Published by Elsevier Inc.

physicianassistant.theclinics.com

It is recommended that all PAs learn about disaster medicine; after reading this issue, you can stay updated by reading the latest news from the Centers for Disease Control and Prevention (https://emergency.cdc.gov) and the National Disaster Medical System (https://www.phe.gov/Preparedness/responders/ndms/Pages/default.aspx).

I hope you enjoy this issue. Our next issue is a little different and will cover Intrinsic Skills for Physician Assistants.

James A. Van Rhee, MS, PA-C
Yale School of Medicine
Yale Physician Assistant Online Program
100 Church Street South, Suite A230
New Haven, CT 06519, USA

E-mail address:
james.vanrhee@yale.edu

Website:
http://www.paonline.yale.edu

REFERENCE

1. American Academy of Physician Assistants. 2018-2019 Policy Manual AAPA 2019. Available at: https://www.aapa.org/download/48096/. Accessed July 1, 2019.

Preface

Disaster Medicine

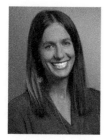

Mary Showstark, MS, PA-C
Editor

Disasters can occur in a moment's notice. Disasters may be caused by terror attacks, man-made accidents, or by Mother Nature. Mass shootings, vehicle attacks, and terror-related bombing and blast injuries are occurring at an alarmingly increasing rate, and providers need to know how to stop the bleed and take care of these patients. Terror attacks may be more sophisticated and include chemical attacks or utilization of pathogens of high consequence. Man-made disasters can occur accidentally, creating radioactively contaminated patients. Mass casualty incidents and natural disasters, such as floods, hurricanes, cyclones, and earthquakes, can leave providers working with limited resources and needing to work utilizing crisis standards of care. Providers must be aware of how to communicate during times of disaster, provide care for vulnerable patients, and most importantly, learn how to cope and care for themselves in these trying times. In this issue, we briefly cover these important elements of working in Disaster Medicine.

Mary Showstark, MS, PA-C
Yale School of Medicine
Physician Assistant Online Program
100 Church Street South, Suite A230
New Haven, CT 06519, USA

E-mail address:
MARY.SHOWSTARK@YALE.EDU

Physician Assist Clin 4 (2019) xiii
https://doi.org/10.1016/j.cpha.2019.07.002
2405-7991/19/© 2019 Published by Elsevier Inc.

physicianassistant.theclinics.com

Crisis Standards of Care

Mary Showstark, MS, PA-C[a],*, Bryan Lovejoy, DNP, FNP-BC[b]

KEYWORDS

- Crisis standards of care • Limited resources • Provider liability
- Mass casualty incidents • Disaster triage • Disaster ethics

KEY POINTS

- History of crisis standards of care.
- Discuss key elements of working with limited resources.
- Briefly discuss triage in MCIs.
- Briefly discuss ethics and working with limited supplies in disaster.

INTRODUCTION

Public health emergencies can take many forms, some are natural, such as hurricanes, wildfires, earthquakes, and tornadoes. Additional events can be caused by people, such as terrorist attacks or acts of war. Examples are nuclear, radiation, and chemical exposures, including dissemination of a drug such as anthrax or a nerve agent such as Novichok. Pandemics, such as influenza, and mass casualty events or incidents are also seen as public health emergencies.[1] Regardless of the cause, these crisis events can overwhelm a health care system. When this occurs, the implementation of crisis standards of care (CSC) designed to optimize health care outcomes is crucial. This article gives a brief overview of CSC as it relates to advanced practice providers (APPs) and offers practical advice applicable to real-world scenarios.

Definition

APPs are all accustomed to standards of care (SOC). An example of this could be surgical care improvement protocols to prevent postsurgical infections. Another example is the chest pain SOC, in which patients who have presumed cardiac chest pain are treated with a set regimen. Additionally, anytime a diabetic patient becomes hypoglycemic institutions have a hypoglycemic protocol that is followed. There are many SOC that APPs are routinely exposed to on a daily basis. SOC are geared to helping APPs in

Disclosure Statement: The authors have nothing to disclose.
[a] Physician Assistant Online Program, Yale School of Medicine, 100 Church Street South, Suite A230, New Haven, CT 06519, USA; [b] Department of Medicine, Northwell Health, Disaster Medical Assistance Team NY4, 300 community drive, Manhasset, NY 11030, USA
* Corresponding author.
E-mail address: MARY.SHOWSTARK@YALE.EDU

Physician Assist Clin 4 (2019) 663–673
https://doi.org/10.1016/j.cpha.2019.06.010
2405-7991/19/© 2019 Elsevier Inc. All rights reserved.

everyday circumstances.[2] However, in times of disaster, an APP may be faced with difficult decisions and may be forced to alter their clinical decision owing to limited supplies, support staff, and high patient volume. Planning must address all of these factors to define appropriate SOC for any situation that constitutes as a crisis. In these situations, SOC have come to be known as CSC. CSC are created to obtain the best health care outcomes in crisis situations.[2] This involves shifting the priority away from routine care to the allocation of medical personnel, supplies, and resources to provide the best care to the greatest number of people effected by the crisis.[1] These protocols allow APPs to continue to perform optimal care under these conditions. CSC occur when there is potential to overwhelm the public health care systems and the rationing of resources is required.

FRAMEWORK

Guidance for establishing CSC for use in crisis situations was developed by the Institute of Medicine (IOM), also known as National Academy of Medicine in 2009 at the request of the US Department of Health and Human Services.[3–5] In 2013, the IOM outlined a toolkit for jurisdictions to identify measurable indicators and triggers. Concepts included in CSC are resource conservation, regional medical staffing, liability protection of providers, pharmaceutical shortages, capacity issues, and standardized infection control, to name a few. The IOM aims to offer these principles: fairness, duty to care, and duty to steward resources; and 4 ethical principles: transparency, consistency, proportionality, and accountability.[1]

The CSC are implemented at the federal, state, and local government levels. This works directly with hospital care, public health workers, out-of-hospital care, emergency services, emergency management, and public safety.[6] It takes provider and community engagement, as well as education and information-sharing, to make this system work. Coordination between federal partners and state health departments and other state agencies help facilitate this effort. Crisis-specific response plans should be in place in terms of call center response and ambulance staffing, and featured at state and local levels (See Figure 2-1 in *Crisis Standards of Care: A Systems Framework for Catastrophic Disaster Response*).[6] Templates exist for state and local government agencies, medical facilities, emergency responders, and community health care delivery systems.[3] The CSC stress that preparation, education and training and especially learning from experience are key factors in handling crisis situations.[7]

CRISIS STANDARDS OF CARE FIELD TRIAGE

Appropriate triage is vital to any crisis operation. It is important to scan crowds of people and locate anyone who is acutely ill and bring them to receive immediate care. Most people who come through triage do not have life-threatening issues and can wait prolonged periods of time, even days if necessary. Triage in a crisis situation is not about customer satisfaction, it is about identifying sick people and saving lives. Medical triage becomes very difficult when the everyday SOC change. Oxygen might not be readily available. Some patients may need decontamination or isolation.

Pandemics may overwhelm the system and surge capacity may exceed the number of staff and the availability of equipment, space, and supplies. For example, President Obama's emergency declaration in response to the H1N1 virus influenza (ie, swine flu) pandemic authorized alternate treatment and triage facilities for patient care.[5] Fortunately, although the potential existed, this strain was not catastrophic to the health care system.

Front-line providers must be able to make life-and-death decisions without the threat of second-guessing to allow them to focus on saving lives and reducing suffering.[1] Triage methods by an APP should be valid, reproducible, and transparent, with fair distribution of scarce or limited resources.[4]

METHODS OF TRIAGE

The simple triage and rapid treatment (START) system is among the most commonly used triage systems that APPs should be aware of (see **Fig. 1**). This triage system is very similar to the sort, assess, lifesaving interventions, treatment

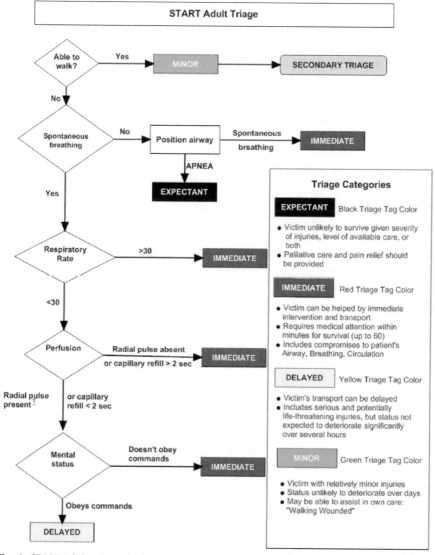

Fig. 1. START adult triage. (*Adapted from* Benson M, Koenig KL SC. Disaster triage: START, then SAVE-a new method of dynamic triage for victims of a catastrophic earthquake. *Prehospital Disaster Med.* 1996;11(2):117-124.)

and/or transport (SALT) system, in which providers tag patients with stickers: black for dead, red for immediate, gray for expectant, yellow for delayed, and green for minimal.[8] This is similar to the move, assess, sort, and send (MASS) system.

There are many different triage systems used, and APPs should keep in mind that there is no single standard triage system. When necessary, APPs should be adaptable with regard to triage.[9,10]

ONGOING ASSESSMENT OF ADMITTED PATIENTS

When working in an inpatient setting during a crisis, an APP may need to rapidly discharge medically stable patients from the ward, making beds and resources available for more critical patients. It can be tremendously challenging to coordinate rapidly with social workers; speech, physical, and occupational therapists; and other specialists to arrange safe transitions out of the hospital. There may even be times when patients may be removed from rooms and placed into the hallways in chairs.

Tools that can be useful in an intensive care unit (ICU) setting are triage scoring systems, such as sequential organ failure assessment (SOFA) and quick SOFA (qSOFA).

A SOFA score assesses the performance of many systems in the body, including neurologic, blood, liver, kidney, and hemodynamics, and assigns a score based on the data obtained in each category (**Table 1**). The higher the SOFA score, the higher the risk for mortality and the greater likelihood of requiring more ICU resources. However, if the SOFA score is low, the patient can likely be discharged to a lower acuity floor or even from the hospital.

The qSOFA score is a bedside triage tool that may identify patients with suspected infection who are at greater risk for a poor outcome outside the ICU. It uses 3 criteria, assigning 1 point for low blood pressure (systolic blood pressure$\leq$100 mm Hg), high respiratory rate ($\geq$22 breaths per minute), or altered mentation (Glasgow coma scale<15).[11] Many states have included some version of the SOFA in their CSC plans.[4,11] APPs should always be continuously evaluating and assessing their patients in order to make sure the best allocation of resources and staffing is being implemented during a crisis.

SPECIAL POPULATIONS

APPs should take into consideration special populations, such as children.[3] The Emergency Medical Services for Children (EMSC) National Pediatric Readiness Project notes that many hospitals and emergency medical services agencies are not equipped to handle children.[12] A report from the EMSC in 2012 stated 89% of children are treated in nonchildren's facilities. They also noted that 6% of all emergency departments had all pediatric equipment on hand, and 90% had 80% of equipment and medications.[13] This was noted when there was no crisis, therefore it can be assumed that these limited resources would be stretched further during a crisis.

An APP should be aware that after a crisis they may have a large number of pediatric patients. APPs can use JumpSTART, which is similar to START but intended for children. If definitive care is not available at a facility, an APP should ensure that they communicate interfacility transfers when the child is stable. Owing to the nature of some crisis situations, the APP may have to take care of populations or perform in specialties they are not typically accustomed to taking care of in their day-to-day role (See JumpSTART algorithm at: https://chemm.nlm.nih.gov/startpediatric.htm).

Table 1
Triage scoring system

Organ System, Measurement	SOFA Score				
	0	**1**	**2**	**3**	**4**
Respiration Pao_2/Fio_2, mm Hg	Normal	<400	<300	<200 (with respiratory support)	<100 (with respiratory support)
Coagulation (Platelets × $10^3/mm^3$)	Normal	<150	<100	<50	<20
Liver Bilirubin, mg/dL (μmol/L)	Normal	1.2–1.9 (20–32)	2.0–5.9 (33–101)	60–11.9 (102–204)	>12.0 (<204)
Cardiovascular Hypotension	Normal	MAP <70 mm Hg	Dopamine ≤5 or dobutamine (any dose)[a]	Dopamine >5 or epinephrine ≤0.1 or norepinephrine ≤0.1	Dopamine >15 or epinephrine >0.1 or norepinephrine >0.1
Central Nervous System Glasgow Coma Score	Normal	13–14	10–12	6–9	<6
Renal Creatinine, mg/dL (μmol/L) or Urine output	Normal	1.2–1.9 (110–170)	2.0–3.4 (171–299)	3.5–4.9 (300–440) or <500 mL/d	>5.0 (>440) or <200 mL/d

Abbreviations: Fio_2, Fraction of inspired oxygen; MAP, Mean arterial pressure.
[a] Adrenergic agents administered for at least 1 hour (doses given are in μg/kg/min).
Adapted from Vincent JL, Moreno R, Takala J, et al. The SOFA (Sepsis-related Organ Failure Assessment) score to describe organ dysfunction/failure. On behalf of the Working Group on Sepsis-Related Problems of the European Society of Intensive Care Medicine Intensive Care Med. 1996 Jul;22(7):707-10; with permission.

PATIENT CARE CONSIDERATIONS

In many crisis situations, most patients seen have low acuity. People might gravitate toward the medical triage area simply because they have no place else to go. Many patients have chronic stable medical conditions, such as hypertension, chronic obstructive pulmonary disease, diabetes, or seizure disorder, but because of the crisis had to leave their homes without their medications. The simple act of renewing medications or distributing them from an APP's pharmacy in a timely manner can prevent patients from decompensating; however, in some situations, the medications may not be available.

When deciding the best course of action for these situations, consider how another APP would deal with the situation under the same circumstances and not how they would deal with it in their normal noncrisis role. For example, if a septic patient presents in a crisis situation and one does not have antibiotics, then one cannot give antibiotics, and any other APP in that situation would not be able to give antibiotics either.

One of best preventive measures an APP can take during a crisis is to stop the spread of infection; this can be done through hand-washing. Handwashing saves lives, even more so then complex medical procedures. Unfortunately, in many of these situations, there is no running water. Hand sanitizers are common alternative but handwashing is the gold standard and should be done whenever possible. It is important to keep environments as clean as possible to decrease the spread of infection.

An additional consideration is the prescription of medications by the APP. The APP needs to make sure to educate patients on the medications. The APP should also weigh whether prescribing will do more harm if the patient runs out of medication. It is important to set appropriate expectations. For example, if a patient has high blood pressure and an APP starts them on medication but they have no one to follow-up with in a month, is there a benefit to starting the medication? Additionally, in crisis situations, APPs will not have access to a laboratory, imaging studies, or basic supplies, and will have to go back to the basic physical examination (**Box 1**).

Supplies

In crisis situations, the APP's initial supplies will come from their employing facility or, if they are working with an organization, from a set cache. Depending on the crisis, supplies may become exhausted. In these cases, an APP should be aware of the Strategic National Stockpile (SNS).

The SNS is the nation's largest supply of potentially lifesaving pharmaceuticals and medical supplies for use in a public health emergency. If local supplies are diminished or depleted, the SNS can be called on.[11] Although this stock pile is a potential resource, it is important to recognize that there are a lot of logistics involved for the SNS to reach a location. There are many steps in this process that can become compromised and these supplies may arrive late or may never arrive.

Box 1
Basics of physical examination

1. History of present illness, OPQRST, or ROS

2. Vital signs

3. HEENT
   Fundoscopic examination or otoscope examination, gross hearing, Weber or Rinne

4. Respiratory-inspection, palpation, lung sounds or percussion-resonance, dullness, respiratory expansion, diaphragmatic excursion

5. CV-inspecting palpating lifts, heaves, thrills, JVD, auscultation (murmurs-sitting, supine, squatting, left lateral decubitus)

6. Abdomen-inspecting, auscultation, percussion (organ size), palpation, Rovsing, psoas, obturator, Murphy, CVA, McBurney, rebound

7. Neurologic: GCS, pronator drift, Finger to Nose, MMSE, pain or dull, CN

8. MSK-ROM, crepitus, warmth

9. Lymph nodes, hernias

10. Sensitive examinations

Abbreviations: CV, cardiac; CVA, costovertebral angle tenderness; GCS, Glasgow Coma Score; HEENNT, head, ears, eyes, nose, neck throat; JVD, jugular venous distention; MSK, Musculoskeletal; OPQRST, onset, pain, palliation, provocation, quality of pain, region and radiation, severity, timing; ROM, Range of Motion; ROS, review of systems.

Another way supplies can arrive is through donations. These supplies can include equipment and medications but must have accepting parties; not be expired; and, internationally, consulates may need to sign off on them. For example, if traveling with large supplies of medications or equipment, such as a defibrillator, the provider should receive a letter of support from the consulate in order to not have supplies detained in customs. Be aware of local laws and procedures to avoid having supplies confiscated or being detained by immigration authorities.

If medications and equipment are not available, the provider must do the best with resources at hand. Strategies to address resource shortages, including preparing, substituting, adapting, conserving, reusing, and reallocating, are provided in "Implications for Care Capacity Continuum for Resources" in *Crisis Standards of Care: A Systems Framework for Catastrophic Disaster Response*[6] and **Box 2**.

STAFFING

Another issue APPs may encounter is working with limited staff. The ability to maintain staffing in a crisis is vital. There may not be a nurse or a technician to help with blood draws or transferring a patient. The APP may have to assume multiple tasks and roles.

Staff may not be able to come in after a disaster. There is the potential that roadways will be blocked. There is the potential that their own home was destroyed or is unsafe. Staff may have young children or elderly relatives who are not safe alone at home.[1,12] Furthermore, depending on the nature of the crisis, there is the possibility that staff will be afraid to be exposed to a major pathogen, such as Ebola. There are many factors, both personal and logistical, that may prevent a provider from showing up to work.

APPs are encouraged to join registries and teams that provide care during public health emergencies. The Emergency System for Advance Registration of Volunteer Health Professionals is a network created by the federal government.[15] Many states have their own medical reserve corps or disaster medical assistance team (DMAT) that stage for disasters. These are effective when advance warning is given and

---

Box 2
Core strategies to address resource shortages

1. Prepare: actions taken before event to minimize resource scarcity (stockpiling of medications)[4]

2. Substitute: use an essentially equivalent device, drug, or personnel for 1 that would usually be available

3. Adapt: use a device, drug, or personnel that are not equivalent but that will provide sufficient care (anesthesia machine for mechanical ventilation, an IM APP in surgery)[14]

4. Conserve: use less of a resource by lowering dosage or changing utilization practices (minimizing use of oxygen-driven nebulizers to conserve oxygen)

5. Reuse: use again items that would normally be single-use items after appropriate disinfection or sterilization

6. Reallocate: restrict or prioritize use of resources to those patients with a better prognosis or greater need

Data from Institute of Medicine (US) Committee on Guidance for Establishing Standards of Care for Use in Disaster Situations; Altevogt BM, Stroud C, Hanson SL (eds), et al. *Guidance for Establishing Crisis Standards of Care for Use in Disaster Situations: A Letter Report,* Washington (DC): National Academies Press (US); 2009.

staging is possible, such as when a hurricane is coming. However, sometimes it may take days for help to arrive. It is always helpful for providers to get involved but providers should also heed warnings from state and federal agencies that may recommend that providers should shelter in place, whether at home or at the hospital.[3]

ETHICS AND LIABILITY

According to the American Medical Association's *Code of Medical Ethics*, providers are obligated to respond during times of a disaster, even if situations are dangerous.[16–18]

However, many APPs might not wish to respond to a crisis because they worry about liability or becoming stuck somewhere, or they may have a concern about their safety or wellbeing. This can be a significant logistical concern to administrators who are trying to provide appropriate staffing. Despite these concerns, fortunately, during times of disaster, many providers opt to respond.[15]

If a disaster occurs at an APP's facility of employment, they should be aware of the facility's disaster protocols and policies. At an individual level, providers should check with their existing employer about how they will be covered if a crisis strikes. An important consideration is will the facility's legal policies or malpractice plan cover an APP working outside the facility? For example, if an APP is assisting with emergency medical services or at a federal DMAT tent, will they be covered? A provider should remember that the Good Samaritan Law (ie, if a provider comes across an accident or an injury, they may assist and be legally covered) does not always apply.

Additional things to consider are the many legal issues that may arise among various organizations, states, counties, or interested parties. Owing to the inconsistency of legality and processes, leaders from varying government organizations and international humanitarian nonprofit groups have asked for increasing transparency, continuity, and consistency among aid groups.[19] One should check with the ministry of health and the volunteer or NGO organization if going overseas (**Box 3**).

A famous case that occurred after Hurricane Katrina is the story of Karen Pou, MD. Dr Pou was working in an inpatient unit and they were not able to evacuate all of her patients. After 4 days, the hospital was finally evacuated, and 45 decomposing corpses were found in the hospital. This was more than any of the other nearby hospitals. Coroners found traces of morphine in the patients and Dr Pou and 2 nurses were accused of euthanasia. Supporters of Dr Pou said that she stayed with her patients while others left

---

Box 3
Examples of federal and state protections

Federal protections
- Uniform Emergency Volunteer Health Practitioners Act
- Public Readiness and Emergency Preparedness (PREP) Act; implementation of covered medical countermeasures
- US Food and Drug Administration issuance of Emergency Use Authorization

State protections
- Emergency laws or regulations tort claims acts
- Emergency management assistance compact
- Intrastate mutual aid legislation

Data from Hodge JG, Hanfling D, Powell TP. Practical, Ethical, and Legal Challenges Underlying Crisis Standards of Care. *J Law, Med Ethics.* 2013. https://doi.org/10.1111/jlme.12039; and *From* Institute of Medicine. 2012. Crisis Standards of Care: A Systems Framework for Catastrophic Disaster Response: Volume 1: Introduction and CSC Framework. Washington, DC: The National Academies Press. https://doi.org/10.17226/13351.

Box 4
What providers can do
Be patient
Be willing to help
Be willing to always do no harm
Recognize that the system is not perfect, that providers improvise, and there are no 100% answers
Get training
Participate in live drills and table top discussions
Participate in simulation

and did what she could for them. She was arrested on 1 count of second-degree murder and 9 counts of conspiracy to commit second-degree murder.[19]

None of the federal regulations provided liability protections for Dr Pou. The federal Emergency Medical Treatment and Active Labor Act (EMTALA) is related to emergency care in the actual emergency room so it did not apply because her patients were inpatient. The Volunteer Protection Act of 1997 provides some immunity to volunteers in disaster settings but did not apply because Dr Pou was not volunteering; she was a paid staff physician.[19] Louisiana's Good Samaritan laws did not apply to on-duty staff physicians.[20,21]

Dr Pou was occupied in lawsuits for several years. The American Medical Academy praised Dr Pou's work despite the charges. Even though she was released of charges, her professional reputation and the traumatic events that she underwent during and after the disaster certainly caused her a substantial amount of stress.

APPs should look into what their state and local laws are in order to know how to function best during a time of a mass casualty event. They should also discuss with their employers what their coverage is in times of disaster. It should be noted that APPs should have not only medical liability insurance but health and evacuation coverage in case they become ill or hurt when working a disaster.[15]

SUMMARY

There is not one set way to perform during a crisis. Providers should take into consideration several factors when in a crisis public health emergency (**Box 4**). Many hospitals and organizations have CSC developed at the county, state, and federal levels. APPs should become familiar with the policies that are available to them in their work environment. Providers should be able to recognize that they may need to function outside of their normal day-to-day role.

Supplies, staffing, and resources are not always readily available. Providers should reuse and reallocate supplies when necessary, and become familiar with triage protocols to help adequately distribute the supplies.

Patience, communication, and adaptability among APPs are key to success. Education exercises and simulation drills are available and providers should participate. APPs who are interested in working in crisis situations should preregister for state reserves and volunteer organizations. Federal careers are also available.

APPs should always remember to be as prepared as possible, adapt as needed, and always strive to do no harm.

REFERENCES

1. Hodge JG, Hanfling D, Powell TP. Practical, ethical, and legal challenges underlying crisis standards of care. J Law Med Ethics 2013. https://doi.org/10.1111/jlme.12039.
2. Leider JP, Debruin D, Reynolds N, et al. Ethical guidance for disaster response, specifically around crisis standards of care: a systematic review. Am J Public Health 2017. https://doi.org/10.2105/AJPH.2017.303882.
3. Murray JS. DISASTER CARE: crisis standards of care: a framework for responding to catastrophic, vol. 112, 2012. Available at: https://www.jstor.org/stable/pdf/23461112.pdf?refreqid=excelsior%3Af5058767a4d2fd6bd7a1e9758986d2ec. Accessed January 16, 2019.
4. Koenig KL, Chin H, Lim S, et al. Crisis standard of care: refocusing health care goals during catastrophic disasters and emergencies 2011. https://doi.org/10.1016/j.jecm.2011.06.003.
5. Lis R, Sakata V, Lien O. How to choose? Using the delphi method to develop consensus triggers and indicators for disaster response, 17. Library (Lond); 2019. https://doi.org/10.1017/dmp.2016.174.
6. Altevogt B. Crisis standards of care: a systems framework for catastrophic disaster response 2012. Atlanta (GA). https://www.phe.gov/coi/Documents/Committee on Guidance for Est SC for Use in Disaster Situations Atlanta Conf.pdf.
7. Firth PG. Standard of care-in sickness and in health and in emergencies, letter to the editor. N Engl J Med 2010;363(14):1378–80.
8. Federal Interagency Committee on EMS. National implementation of the model uniform core criteria for mass casualty incident triage, 2014. Available at: https://asprtracie.hhs.gov/technical-resources/resource/4673/national-implementation-of-the-model-uniform-core-criteria-for-mass-casualty-incident-triage-a-report-of-the-ficems.
9. Lerner EB, Schwartz RB, McGovern JE. Prehospital triage for mass casualties 2015. Available at: https://www.emergencymedicine.pitt.edu/sites/default/files/4.2 Prehospital Triage for Mass Casualties_0.pdf. Accessed March 15, 2019.
10. Newport Beach CFD. START Support Services. Available at: http://citmt.org/Start/thanks.htm.
11. Gostin LO, Hanfling D. National preparedness for a catastrophic emergency. JAMA 2009;302(21):2365.
12. Dahl Grove D. Pediatric preparedness: children's hospitals preparation for disasters. Curr Treat Options Pediatr 2017;3(3):246–53.
13. Weik T. Emergency medical services for children. Improving the emergency care system for America's children. U.S. Department of Health and Human Services: HRSA. Available at: https://www.ems.gov/pdf/nemsac/march2012/HRSA_EMS_for_Children-Tasmeen_Weik-March2012_NEMSAC.pdf. Accessed March 10, 2019.
14. New York State Department of Health and New York State task force on life and the law update ventilator allocation guidelines. 2015. Available at: https://www.health.ny.gov/press/releases/2015/2015-11   25_ventilator_allocation_guidelines.htm. Accessed March 20, 2019.
15. Schultz CH, Annas GJ. Altering the standard of care in disasters-unnecessary and dangerous. Ann Emerg Med 2012;59:191–5.
16. AMA. Physicians' responsibilities in disaster response & preparedness. 2010. Available at: https://www.ama-assn.org/delivering-care/ethics/physicians-responsibilities-disaster-response-preparedness. Accessed March 20, 2019.

17. AMA. Physicians' responsibilities in disaster preparedness. Available at: https://journalofethics.ama-assn.org/article/ama-code-medical-ethics-opinion-physician-duty-treat/2010-06. Accessed March 10, 2019.
18. Association AM. Opinion 9.067 physician obligation in disaster preparedness and response. Code of medical ethics. Available at: http://www.ama-assn.org/ama/pub/physician-resources/medical-ethics/code-medical-ethics/opinion9067.shtml. Accessed March 20, 2019.
19. Schultz CH, Annas GJ. In reply. Ann Emerg Med 2012;60(5):670–1.
20. Fink S. No title. Five days at Memorial. 2014. Available at: http://www.sherifink.net/dr-anna-pou. Accessed March 13, 2019.
21. Charpentier C. Grand jury refuses to indict Dr. Anna Pou. 2007. Available at: http://blog.nola.com/times-picayune/2007/07/grand_jury_refuses_to_indict_d.html. Accessed March 20, 2019.

Vulnerable Populations in Disaster

Residence, Resilience, and Resources

Ralph R. Stanton Jr, MA[a],*,
Amelia M. Duran-Stanton, PhD, DSc, MPAS, PA-C[b]

KEYWORDS

- Disaster • Residence • Resilience • Resources • Social vulnerability
- Spatial analysis

KEY POINTS

- According to the Centers for Disease Control and Prevention (CDC), vulnerable populations are the following: (1) have difficulty communicating, (2) difficulty accessing medical care, (3) may need help maintaining independence, (4) require constant supervision, and (5) may need help accessing transportation.
- Social vulnerability is more than hazards and risks—it includes complex problems with residence, resilience, and resources linked to geopolitical systems and historical structures.
- The CDC and other medical organizations promote the use of spatial analysis and thematic maps to visualize vulnerable populations.
- Thematic maps may be produced by the CDC's Social Vulnerability Index to visualize vulnerable populations within the United States.
- To reduce social vulnerability, people need help with residence, resilience, and resources to deal with everything from socioeconomic status to disabilities, housing, and transportation issues.

INTRODUCTION

The World Health Organization defines vulnerability as "the degree to which population, individual or organization is unable to anticipate, cope with, resist, and recover from the impact of disasters."[1] According to the Centers for Disease Control and Prevention (CDC), vulnerable populations are the following: (1) have difficulty communicating, (2) difficulty accessing medical care, (3) may need help maintaining independence, (4) require constant supervision, and (5) may need help accessing transportation.[2] Medical professionals must have a great understanding of the disease burden of vulnerable populations such as those involving pregnant women, children,

Disclosure Statement: No disclosures.
[a] 2338 TX-1604 Loop #120, San Antonio, TX 78248, USA; [b] Installation Management Command, G1, R2/ASAP Division, Bldg 2261, 2405 Gun Shed Road, JBSA-Fort Sam Houston, TX 78234 USA
* Corresponding author.
E-mail address: ralph.stanton37@gmail.com

the elderly, malnourished, ill, and immunocompromised. Medical professionals require an understanding of vulnerable populations in disaster in terms of their residence, resilience, and resources. Disasters displace people, especially vulnerable populations burdened by 5 faces of oppression: (1) exploitation, (2) marginalization, (3) cultural imperialism, (4) powerlessness, and (5) violence.[3–5] Geopolitics, globalization, and history are linked to health and well-being, as well as positions of power in different places throughout the world.[4,6,7]

SOCIAL VULNERABILITY

Social vulnerability is more than hazards and risks—it includes complex problems with residence, resilience, and resources linked to geopolitical systems and historical structures. *Residence* implies both a habitat and the way power is distributed over space and time. *Resilience* is thought of as the power to bounce back from crisis, but this depends on the resources that are available before, during, and after disaster response takes place. *Resources*, like power and resilience, are managed over space and time, which is why spatial analysis and thematic maps may be used to visualize vulnerable populations as a whole.[8–12]

VISUALIZING VULNERABLE POPULATIONS: THEMATIC MAPS

The CDC and other medical organizations promote the use of spatial analysis and thematic maps to visualize vulnerable populations.[2,8,12–14] Thematic maps may be produced by the CDC's Social Vulnerability Index (SVI) to visualize vulnerable populations within the United States. For instance, to tell a story about vulnerable populations, thematic maps may be designed to visualize overall social vulnerability (ie, emotional and social factors) and compare the complexity of it with 4 themes (ie, **Fig. 1**) in a specific place (ie, physical and environmental factors), such as the United States Census tracts within Bexar County, Texas (**Figs. 2** and **3**). Looking at the different thematic maps, there are darker and lighter colors to indicate the location of vulnerable populations within the larger landscape of Bexar County, where the City of San Antonio is located. Moreover, the themes and variables are weighed to provide an overall view of vulnerable populations that may be compared with 4 *Others*: (1) socioeconomic, (2) household composition and disability, (3) minority status and language, and (4) housing and transportation. Thematic maps, derived from geospatial data to create the CDC's SVI 2016 spatial analysis of Bexar County (see **Figs. 2** and **3**), provide reference points to help medical professionals make some important decisions about vulnerable populations.

Thematic maps, such as those of Bexar County, Texas (see **Figs. 2** and **3**), theoretically work as reference points to visualize vulnerable populations over space and time (ie, Bexar County's geospatial data from 2016 SVI), where the whole is other than the 4 themes and 15 variables (see **Fig. 1**). There is evidence from disaster scholarship that people need resilience and resources to reduce social vulnerability and increase survival rates when they are exposed to hazards and risks, which is why emergency managers are trying to use geospatial data to educate stakeholders in private, public, and nonprofit organizations to understand responder communications, wherefrom people are figuratively and literally coming (over space and time).[8,9,11–13,15,16] These maps tell us where people face socioeconomic problems, such as education and employment, that may prevent them from getting access to care and other resources associated with survival, such as income, insurance, and savings for emergency situations. They also inform us of problems faced by people such as age, disabilities, and risks associated with lives in a

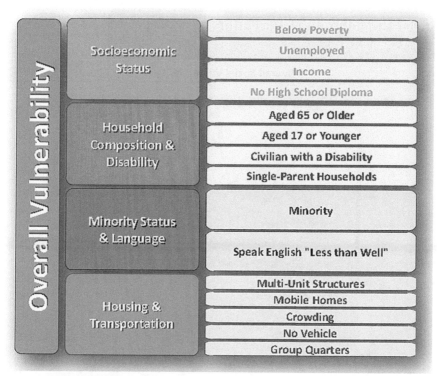

Fig. 1. Overall social vulnerability and 4 theme variables. (*Data from* Center for Disease Control and Prevention (CDC)'s Agency for Toxic Substances and Disease Registry (ATSDR). SVI 2016 Documentation - 1/24/2018.; 2018. https://svi.cdc.gov/Documents/FactSheet/SVIFactSheet.pdf.)

single-parent household—all of these variables will frequently limit access to messages delivered by electronic devices and social media. These maps tell us where ethnic groups and minority individuals are located, as well as people who may not understand communications limited to English, and inform us about people's problems with housing and transportation, where more people living in group quarters, low-income housing, mobile parks, overcrowded facilities, and taller buildings in urbanized areas (such as homeless people, prisoners, soldiers, students, and transient workers) are more vulnerable, especially when they do not own a vehicle to evacuate themselves from an area that will be struck by a disaster.

These maps are reference points. They point out where vulnerable populations reside. They point out behavior patterns with resilience, such as who goes where when disaster strikes and local resources are overwhelmed. They point out which resources are available and where they move to over space and time. Thus, to understand vulnerable populations during a disaster, it is important to acknowledge social vulnerability and study issues associated with residence, resilience, and resources over space and time to reduce social vulnerability—defined by the CDC as a community's capacity to prepare for and respond to hazardous events, whereby social factors affect that community's ability to prevent human suffering and financial loss.[2] Medical professionals need to know these factors to enable them to plan and mitigate when serving in all phases of the disaster. Vulnerable populations have a higher likelihood of suffering from injury, disease, or death.[1,5,9,11,17–19]

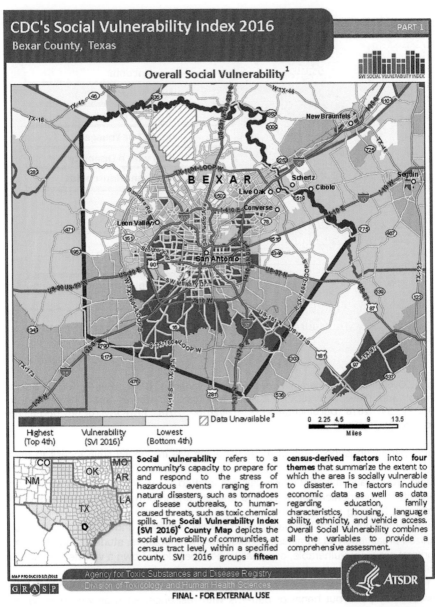

Fig. 2. Overall social vulnerability. (*Data from* CDC's Social Vulnerability Index: Bexar County, Texas. Available at: https://svi.cdc.gov/.)

RESIDENCE: HABITAT AND STATE OF POWER

Residence may be thought of in 2 ways. First, it is a habitat—the location where somebody resides. Second, it is a state of power—as in the rights of citizens and residents to be protected by individuals and institutions. For instance, one may reside in the United States physically and environmentally, but without the legal residence there is difficulty in getting access to health care benefits when exposed to hazards and

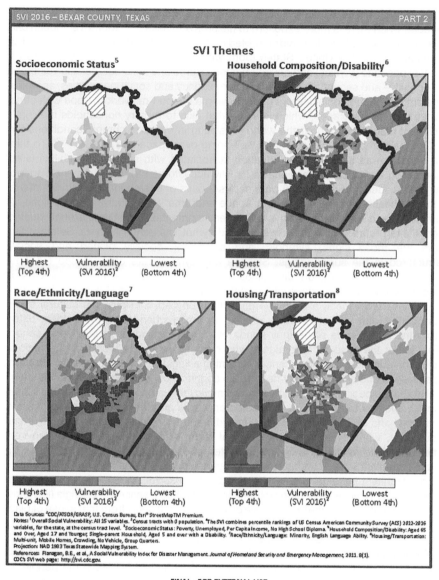

Fig. 3. Four SVI themes. (*Data from* CDC's Social Vulnerability Index: Bexar County, Texas. Available at: https://svi.cdc.gov/.)

risks, such as Latinos living in North Carolina as migrant and seasonal workers in the agriculture industry, or indigenous people in Ecuador who migrate to an area where there is an active volcano and find employment in the geological-tourism industry.[17,20] In both cases, exploitation is interrelated to migration that exposes people to physical hazards and risks, as well as socioeconomic opportunities to travel abroad and learn different languages. Latinos (of any race) throughout the United States are usually earning lower incomes in comparison with other men and women with similar educational backgrounds; and graduate or professional degrees usually contribute to higher incomes that increase access to care, continuity of care, and quality of care, which is needed when there is more exposure to hazards and risks.[18,21] Moreover, health care insurance is linked to Medicaid and Medicare programs tied into residency, so that Latinos living in the United States (both with and without documentation) are not only exposed to physical and environmental hazards and risks but are also vulnerable to cognitive and semiotic factors linked to residency and social inequalities, as well as the emotional and social factors of not having a support network to cope with stress when they are displaced, which is somewhat akin to military households moving to different places throughout the world—resulting in multiple, chronic conditions that affect the complexity of health and well-being over space and time.[18,22–25] To think of residence as a geopolitical situation (associated with social vulnerability) is not something a medical professional is usually accustomed to, but it may help to look at how residency is linked to 6 parameters/3 pairs of interconnected factors interrelated to health and well-being over space and time: (1) cognitive and semiotic, (2) emotional and social, and (3) physical and environmental. Cognitive is an individual/internal interpretation of signs, symbols, and symptoms, among others. Semiotic factors are those signs, symbols, and symptoms socially placed and socially structured in the surroundings. Signage and symbols are often placed for those who are literate and without disabilities. Vulnerable populations will often lack insight into the semiotic structures, such as English-language signs and texts, which may not help those who speak a language other than English. Similarly, the cultural codes associated with semiotics, such as saluting a flag when you are a soldier, differs from the way people place their hands over the heart, which is learned in school. This is not the case for a foreigner who may not know the words to the national anthem, much less the significance of saluting a flag. When health care organizations place signs and symbols, they need to be cognitive of how people feel about them.

Residence begins with cognitive and semiotic factors associated with social vulnerability, such as the detection of hazards and risks and the documentation of signs, symbols, and symptoms. Residence includes the way individuals interpret their surroundings, whereby emotional and social factors transform physical and environmental spaces into a sense of place rooted in experiences and feelings about the architectural structures and surrounding landscapes.[26–28] Residencies include some of the architectural structures and real property in surrounding landscapes, such as the way a flag invokes a patriotic experience, as well as a sense of nostalgia (ie, homesickness) that occurs when people are displaced or drift away from that sense of place to go somewhere else to settle and struggle with a new habitat.[29,30] "Residual scripts," described by Stephen Cairns to introduce *Drifting: Architecture and Migrancy* (2004), helps to understand vulnerable populations in disaster as both an ontologic displacement and a physical movement from one place to another where some people are settled, which becomes unsettling to a group when a strange group migrates into the settlement:

Regarding architecture and migrancy, what is it that brings these terms together in this way? The two terms activate opposite meanings, one being associated with the groundedness of buildings, the constitution of places, and the delimitation of territories, the other with uprootedness, mobility, and the transience of individuals and groups of people. Yet so neat is the opposition between the terms that in Western thought they were often brought together as counterparts within a more general binary relation. This binary relation privileged such principles as settlement, stability, and permanence over those of movement, flux, and fluidity. Migrancy, in its various enforced and voluntary forms, was aligned with the suspect qualities of movement, and so came to be the unfortunate exception to a more general principle of settlement. Within this logic, the migrant was ascribed kinship with the nomad, the Scythian, the gypsy, the wild man, and other figures that haunted the imagination of the settled citizen.[29]

Residents that settle in a community and are continuously exposed to disasters will sometimes become accustomed to living with hazards and risks—these are disaster subcultures or at-risk subpopulations that will experience more social vulnerability because they will often ignore or do not have a means to prepare or respond to alerts and warnings when instructed to evacuate or shelter-in-place.[9,31,32] For instance, disaster subcultures included people who ignored mandatory evacuations when wildfires struck southern California: "As the population in southern California has increased, so has the number of people who have chosen to reside in, or adjacent to, lands prone to wildfire."[32] Sundry reasons why they were unsure, unlikely, or unwilling to evacuate included: they wanted to stay and their protect homes, they felt that their property was safe (thanks to wildfire prevention measures); they would use their own judgment in evacuating; they felt that evacuation was "overkill" by public officials; they felt concerned about their pets or animals; they worried about valuables; and they felt that evacuation was inconvenient.[32] To address these issues, it is recommended that public officials reach out to residents who are unlikely to evacuate and collaborate with local homeowner groups to provide information about pet-friendly places (ie, shelters, hotels, motels), availability of fireproof safes and containers to protect valuables, measures for shelter-in-place, and request the signing of waivers to document how their property is unsafe and that failing to evacuate jeopardizes their own safety and the safety of first responders.[32]

Similarly, people who settle in one place are accustomed to hazards and risks, especially when they have been exposed to several disasters and survived. Thus, disaster subcultures and vulnerable subgroups include people living in communities that are so familiar with disastrous hazards and risks (eg, earthquakes, hurricanes, floods, and tornadoes) "that they become less concerned about the severity of the threat even when a warning is issued."[31] This was what happened with many disaster subcultures during hurricanes Katrina and Maria that destroyed lives and ruined landscapes in Louisiana and Puerto Rico. Hurricane Katrina was a category 5 tropical storm and New Orleans was one of the worst affected because of its geographic location below sea level and protection by levees.[33–35] The vulnerable populations, even with evacuation orders, remained in order to protect their property or lack of affordability to leave. Hurricane Maria's destruction affected Puerto Rico's fragile electric grid and the island already had pre-existing infrastructure challenges, so public health and the health system worsened owing to conditions of the infrastructure.[33,35–41] Moreover, because health care coverage was a problem for people in both locations (some people would use emergency departments for medical prescriptions and routine care) before the disasters, pre-existing conditions worsened over space and time in the postdisaster phases of response and recovery.[5,18,35,36,38,40] Thus, people who had learned to live without medical services and survived previous natural disasters (ie, disaster subcultures and vulnerable subgroups) suffered more when a more severe situation emerged from catastrophic incidents to destroy emergency departments and first-responder capabilities.[31,42]

Thematic maps, such as those used by the CDC, help to visualize where vulnerable populations are located, and these maps may be useful tools for medical professionals. They may be used to reach out to residents and reduce social vulnerability, which is defined by the CDC as follows: "Social vulnerability refers to the resilience of communities when confronted by external stresses on human health, stresses such as natural or human-caused disasters, or disease outbreaks."[2] Whereas a two-variable simplicity of hazards and risks is the traditional way of viewing vulnerability, there has been a paradigm shift to reduce social vulnerability with resilience, which is more of an organized complexity than a random, disorganized complexity. Without an adequate supply of preventive and routine forms of medicine (such as influenza, polio, and rubella vaccines) before a disaster occurs, the proximity of people enclosed in a residence (such as a temporary shelter for displaced individuals) increases exposure to hazards and risks that would otherwise not have existed, exemplifying an organized complexity versus the disorganized complexity of exposure to uncertain phenomena (such as an Ebola outbreak).[43,44]

RESILIENCE

Resilience is a hierarchy of response mechanisms to manage resources, which differs from traditional views about vulnerable populations adapting to environments with biological and cultural functions. For instance, medical anthropologists defined adaptation as "changes, modifications, and variations enabling a person or group to survive in a given environment," but resilience was defined as a "new construct," denoting "the flexibility of humans to respond to problems through a hierarchy of response potentials, some genetic and physiologic, others behavioral and cultural."[15] Vulnerability was defined as "a function of the population's exposure to hazardous conditions and its adaptive capacity" for addressing, planning, and adapting to that exposure.[15] Social vulnerability is linked to resilience, which is tied into the way people interpret their built environments (ie, their homes and possessions and property) to develop a sense of place (ie, their emotional and social connections with physical and environmental spaces). Health care professionals need to know the culture and circumstances of the disasters they support to obtain a better understanding of the community's needs and also what a community can provide to help itself recover from the devastation. A better understanding of the community's historical behavioral and cultural norms even in vulnerable populations provides the health care professionals assistance in identifying which types of resources to provide.

RESOURCES

To reduce social vulnerability, residents need resilience, which includes response mechanisms to manage resources within medical systems that are disrupted when disaster strikes and plans fail, although there are different perspectives about resilience interrelated with space and time.[10,15,45,46] To reach out to vulnerable populations in disaster who reside in a specific place, these populations need to know that those responsible for their health and well-being are willing to provide resources, such as human resources (eg, professionals and volunteers), informational resources (eg, media and messages), and logistical resources (eg, supplies and transportation). Without resources, resilience is diminished and social vulnerability increases. Health care professionals can assist in determining the languages for which interpreters and translators will be needed, and determine requirements in coordination with the American Red Cross in gathering logistical resources.

SUMMARY

Medical professionals must consider vulnerable populations' residence, resilience, and available resources. Medical professionals need to know where the vulnerable populations are located by using available resources such as thematic maps. Medical professionals must consider the resilience of the vulnerable populations to assess their response mechanisms to manage resources and how adaptable they are, based on their location and cultural norms. Because social vulnerability is directly linked to resilience, medical professionals must have a clear understanding of how this also affects where the vulnerable populations choose to live, which resources they have, and which resources they will need when disaster strikes as well as how to mitigate, plan, and assist when required. To reduce social vulnerability, vulnerable populations need help with residence, resilience, and resources to deal with everything from housing and transportation issues to socioeconomic status.

REFERENCES

1. World Health Organization (WHO). WHO: Vulnerable Groups. Environmental health in emergencies and disasters: a practical guide. 2002. Available at: https://www.who.int/environmental_health_emergencies/vulnerable_groups/en/?fbclid=IwAR1eg4DQlpa-Z2bVgWLnKMOhskFdFZXROGYcsqPdj9_qQdyyt8H2JnMgpFg. Accessed April 1, 2019.
2. Center for Disease Control and Prevention (CDC)'s Agency for Toxic Substances and Disease Registry (ATSDR). SVI 2016 documentation—1/24/2018.; 2018. Available at: https://svi.cdc.gov/Documents/FactSheet/SVIFactSheet.pdf. Accessed March 15, 2019.
3. Arnold M. Disaster reconstruction and risk management for poverty reduction. J Int Aff 2006;59(2):269.
4. Young IM. Justice and the politics of difference. Princeton (NJ): Princeton University Press; 1990.
5. Hoffman S. Preparing for disaster: protecting the most vulnerable in emergencies case research paper series in legal studies. 2008;(April):1491-1547. Available at: http://ssrn.com/abstract=1268277CASEWESTERNRESERVEUNIVERSITYhttp://ssrn.com/abstract=1268277http://www.law.case.edu/ssrn. Accessed March 15, 2019.
6. Geopolitics: geography and strategy. In: Gray CS, Sloan G, editors. Portland (OR): Frank Cass; 1999.
7. Krieger N. Epidemiology and the people's health: theory and context. 1st edition. New York: Oxford University Press; 2011.
8. Flanagan BE, Hallisey EJ, Adams E, et al. Measuring community vulnerability to natural and anthropogenic hazards: the Centers for Disease Control and Prevention's Social Vulnerability Index. J Environ Health 2018;80(10):34–7.
9. Ramisetty-Mikler S, Mikler AR, O'Neill M, et al. Conceptual framework and quantification of population vulnerability for effective emergency response planning. J Emerg Manag 2015;13(3):227.
10. Walker B, Westley F. Perspectives on resilience to disasters across sectors and cultures. Ecol Soc 2011;16(2). https://doi.org/10.5751/ES-04070-160204.
11. Dolan G, Messen D. Social vulnerability: an emergency managers' planning tool. J Emerg Manag 2013;10(3):161.
12. Alexander D, Barton AH, Boin A, et al. In: Perry RW, Quarantelli EL, editors. What is a disaster? New answers to old questions, vols. I-II. Bloomington (IN): Xlibris; 2005. p. 1–442.
13. Tate E. Social vulnerability index. Ann Assoc Am Geogr 2013;103(3):526–43.
14. CDC's Social Vulnerability Index: Bexar County, Texas. Available at: https://svi.cdc.gov/Documents/CountyMaps/2016/Texas/Texas2016_Bexar.pdf. Accessed March 15, 2019.

15. McElroy A, Townsend PK. Medical anthropology in ecological perspective. Boulder (CO): Westview Press; 2009.
16. Wexler MD, MPH B, Smith MD, et al. Disaster response and people experiencing homelessness: addressing challenges of a population with limited resources. J Emerg Manag 2015;13(3):195.
17. Montz BE, Allen TR, Monitz GI. Systemic trends in disaster vulnerability: migrant and seasonal farm workers in North Carolina. Risk Hazards Crisis Public Policy 2011;2(1):82–98.
18. Phibbs S, Kenney C, Rivera-Munoz G, et al. The inverse response law: theory and relevance to the aftermath of disasters. Int J Environ Res Public Health 2018; 15(5):916.
19. Bethel JW, Foreman AN, Burke SC. Disaster preparedness among medically vulnerable populations. Am J Prev Med 2011;40(2):139–43.
20. Heggie TW. Geotourism and volcanoes: health hazards facing tourists at volcanic and geothermal destinations. Travel Med Infect Dis 2009;7(5):257–61.
21. Julian T, Kominski R. Education and synthetic work-life earnings estimates American community survey reports. 2011;(September):1-14. Available at: https://www.census.gov/prod/2011pubs/acs-14.pdf. Accessed March 15, 2019.
22. Méndez-Lázaro P, Muller-Karger FE, Otis D, et al. A heat vulnerability index to improve urban public health management in San Juan, Puerto Rico. Int J Biometeorol 2018;62(5):709–22.
23. Institute of Medicine. Gulf war and health physiologic, psychologic, and psychosocial effects of deployment-related stress, vol. 6. Washington, DC: National Academies Press; 2008. https://doi.org/10.17226/11922.
24. National Academies of Sciences, Engineering and Medicine. Gulf war and health generational health effects of serving in the Gulf war, vol. 11. Washington, DC: National Academies Press; 2018. https://doi.org/10.17226/25162.
25. Topolski S. Understanding health from a complex systems perspective. J Eval Clin Pract 2009;15(4):749–54.
26. Jackson JB, Lewis PF, Lowenthal D, et al. In: Meinig DW, editor. The interpretation of ordinary landscapes. New York: Oxford University Press; 1979. p. 1–247.
27. Rasmussen SE. Experiencing architecture. 24th Print. Cambridge (MA): MIT Press; 1959.
28. Yi-Fu T. Space and place: the perspective of experience. 7th Pr. Minneapolis (MN): University of Minnesota Press; 1977.
29. Abbas A, Austin M, Cairns S, et al. Drifting: architecture and migrancy. In: Cairns S, editor. New York: Routledge; 2004.
30. Thomas CL, editor. Taber's cyclopedic medical dictionary. 18th edition. Philadelphia: F.A. Davis Company; 1997. p. 1310.
31. Sellnow DD, Sellnow TL. The IDEA model for effective instructional risk and crisis communication by emergency managers and other key spokespersons. J Emerg Manag 2019;17(1):67.
32. Roberson BS, Peterson D, Parsons RW. Attitudes on wildfire evacuation: exploring the intended evacuation behavior of residents living in two Southern California communities. J Emerg Manag 2013;10(5):335.
33. Long B. 2017 hurricane season FEMA after-action report. 2017. 2018:65. Available at: https://www.fema.gov/media-library-data/1533643262195-6d13983394 49ca85942538a1249d2ae9/2017FEMAHurricaneAARv20180730.pdf. Accessed March 15, 2019.
34. Quarantelli EL. Catastrophes are different from disasters: some implications for crisis planning and managing drawn from Katrina. Issue Br Publ June 11,

2006 Retrieved from Soc Sci Res Counc. 2006:1-6. http://understandingkatrina.ssrc.org/Quarantelli/.

35. Vick K. Lessons from Maria. Time 2018. Available at: https://www.magzter.com/US/Time-Inc/Time/Journals/303584. Accessed March 15, 2019.

36. O'Loughlin MJ. The death toll in Puerto Rico after Hurricane Maria could be 70 times higher than official count 2017. Available at: https://www.americamagazine.org/politics-society/2018/05/30/puerto-rico-death-toll-could-be-70-times-higher-originally-reported.

37. Kishore N, Marqués D, Mahmud A, et al. Mortality in Puerto Rico after Hurricane Maria. N Engl J Med 2018;379(2):162–70.

38. Roman J. Hurricane Maria: a preventable humanitarian and health care crisis unveiling the Puerto Rican dilemma. Ann Am Thorac Soc 2018;15(3):293–5.

39. Morgan R, Prewitt Diaz JO. Editor's note: Hurricane Maria, personal and collective suffering, and psychosocial support as a cross-cutting intervention. J Trop Psychol 2017;7(5):e5.

40. Santos-Burgoa C, Sandberg J, Suárez E, et al. Differential and persistent risk of excess mortality from Hurricane Maria in Puerto Rico: a time-series analysis. Lancet Planet Health 2018;2(11):e478–88.

41. Rodríguez-Díaz CE. Maria in Puerto Rico: natural disaster in a colonial archipelago. Am J Public Health 2018;108(1):30–2.

42. Runkle JD, Brock-Martin A, Karmaus W, et al. Secondary surge capacity: a framework for understanding long-term access to primary care for medically vulnerable populations in disaster recovery. Am J Public Health 2012;102(12):24–33.

43. Benavides AD, McEntire D, Carlson EK. The logic of uncertainty and executive discretion in decision making: the Dallas-Fort Worth Metroplex Ebola response. JPMSP 2017;24(1):2.

44. Sumter JL, Goodrich-Doctor A, Roberts J, et al. Twenty-first century emergency response efforts of the Commissioned Corps of the US Public Health Service. J Emerg Manag 2018;16(5):311–9.

45. Sledge D, Thomas HF. From disaster response to community recovery: nongovernmental entities, government, and public health. Am J Public Health 2019;109(3):437–44.

46. Jones N, Greenberg N, Wessely S. No plans survive first contact with the enemy: flexibility and improvisation in disaster mental health. Psychiatry 2011;70(4):361–5.

Responder Communications in Disaster: Is Less Really More?

Ralph R. Stanton Jr, MA[a],*,
Amelia M. Duran-Stanton, PhD, DSc, MPAS, PA-C[b]

KEYWORDS

- Convergence behavior • Emergency management • Public health • Social media

KEY POINTS

- Medical professionals in clinic and hospital settings need to account for convergence behavior to disrupt responder communications in disaster, especially when there is a mass casualty situation that overwhelms local resources.
- It is key to acknowledge the art of *emergency management* (ie, *mitigation, preparedness, response,* and *recovery*) linked to different types of *improvisation* (ie, *reproductive, adaptive,* and *creative*).
- Medical professions should collect data, identify resources, and share information with internal stakeholders to facilitate dialogue about key messages, situation reports, and social media.
- It is important to define stakeholders and design a communications strategy to create key messages and viably use the IDEA Model to distribute key messages.
- Convergence behavior (ie, spontaneous movement of human, informational, and logistical resources over space and time) affects responder communications (in disaster medicine).

INTRODUCTION: "IS LESS REALLY MORE?"

"Less is more" versus "less is a bore." These 2 opposing adages are applicable to architecture and art, as well as responder communications (in disaster medicine). "Less is more" is frequently attributed to the Bauhaus designer and teacher, Ludwig Mies van der Rohe (1886–1969), whereas "less is a bore" is a postmodern counterpoint attributed to Robert Venturi (1925–2018), the author of *Complexity and Contradiction in Architecture* (1966).[1(p184)] Although his modernist style and Bauhaus works in the first half of the twentieth century (marking today's landscapes and skylines) are still revered for cubist simplicity (creating an illusion of steel skeletons and glass boxes), Mies van der Rohe would also say, "God is in the detail."[1–4] In the second half of

Disclosure Statement: No disclosures.
[a] 2338 TX-1604 Loop #120, San Antonio, TX 78248, USA; [b] Installation Management Command, G1, R2/ASAP Division, Bldg 2261, 2405 Gun Shed Road, JBSA-Fort Sam Houston, TX 78234, USA
* Corresponding author.
E-mail address: ralph.stanton37@gmail.com

the twentieth century, "less is a bore" emerged from critical thoughts from Venturi and others to explain how electronic devices and graphic designs transformed post-modern architecture and poststructuralist landscapes when popular culture was directly placed onto built environments, exemplified in *Learning from Las Vegas: The forgotten symbolism of architectural form* (1972).[1–3,5]

RESPONDER COMMUNICATIONS (IN DISASTER MEDICINE)

Likewise, responder communications (in disaster medicine) have been transformed by the built environment, as well as twenty-first century electronic devices, social media, and technological advances that have helped to improve survival rates, yet there are many individuals and institutions that are not taking advantage of this technology to collect data, facilitate dialogue, and share information interrelated to art of emergency management (ie, mitigation, preparedness, response, recovery).[6–13]

SOCIAL MEDIA AND SOCIAL NETWORKING PLATFORMS

Social media and social networking platforms, such as Facebook, Twitter, YouTube, Instagram, Pinterest, and LinkedIn, have increased in popularity since their infancy, some less than 2 decades ago, such as the terrorist attacks of September 11, 2001 (aka 9/11) that transformed responder communications throughout New York City and other places in the United States; and this was followed by bombings in both Boston, Massachusetts (April 15, 2013) and Austin, Texas (March 2018).[14–19] To deal with explosive acts of violence linked to the adage "whatever bleeds, leads," responders use technological advances in both audio and visual forms of communication, as well as geographic information systems to produce maps for the purposes of both emergency management and homeland security—an invaluable tool for those responding to school shootings, suicides, and other manmade hazards, as well as natural disasters (ie, earthquakes, hurricanes, tornadoes, etc.)[20]

CONVERGENCE BEHAVIOR: IMPROVING RESPONDER COMMUNICATIONS

To improve responder communications (in disaster medicine), it is imperative that medical professionals account for *convergence behavior*—a problem with social control due to the spontaneous, mass movement of human, informational, and logistical resources into a disaster-struck area, whereby expected and unexpected resources will arrive over space and time during the uncertain period between response and recovery phases of emergency management.

There is the phenomenon of "convergence behavior" as people are attracted to disasters for a variety of reasons. Such volunteers can provide needed manpower for disaster operations if integrated into the existing emergency management system but may interfere with the operations of response agencies if they are not organized and used effectively.[21–26]

This was exemplified by the terrorist attacks of 9/11 when both laypersons and medical professionals were well intentioned in their attempts to assist first responders, but the convergence behavior disrupted health care operations.[22]

SIMPLICITY

The idea of "less is more" may include another euphemism—the *KISS Principle: keep it simple, stupid.*[27] There are arguments that simplistic key messages must be distributed by spokespersons who are credible and trustworthy, especially when disaster strikes and local resources are overwhelmed and texts are unfamiliar to recepients.[13,18,28] These messages will occur while people in the private, public, and nonprofit sectors try to manage emergency situations as plans fail, social constructs are disrupted, and people become mentally and physically displaced from their home-lands, their houses, their possessions, and their sense of place tied into familiar spaces. This results in different types of improvisation, such as what happened shortly after 9/11, when responders were overwhelmed by something unimaginable:

In reproductive improvisation, improvisers recreate an existing capacity; in adaptive improvisation, they amend an existing capacity to match changing demands, produc-ing a new system, and in creative improvisation they create an entirely new capacity in the absence of an existing model. All of these forms occur under tight time constraints and with pressing demands for action.[16(p326)]

After 9/11, people wanted simple solutions to plan for complex problems asso-ciated with emergency management and responder communications. On the surface, this seemed possible, but emergency management requires different types improvisation due to the uncertainty associated with drastic changes over space and time. Perhaps this "less is more" aphorism is more complex than the KISS principle tries to imply—manifest in a Taoist folktale to introduce *The Illustrated Art of War*:

ACCORDING TO AN OLD STORY, a lord of ancient China once asked his physician, a member of a family of healers, which of them was most skilled in the art.

The physician, whose reputation was such that his name became synonymous with medical science in China, replied:

My eldest brother sees the spirit of sickness and removes it before it takes shape, so his name does not get out of the house.

My elder brother cures sickness when it is still extremely minute, so his name does not get out of the neighborhood.

As for me, I puncture veins, prescribe potions, and massage skin, so from time to time my name gets out and is heard among the lords.[29(p9)]

Less becomes more. Less *this* results in more of *that*. Less preventive medicine (represented by the eldest brother in the Taoist folktale) equates to more primary care (represented by the elder brother in the Taoist folktale). Less primary care equa-tes to more expensive prescriptions and specialized treatments, such as surgical in-terventions (represented by the famous physician associated with medical science in the Taoist folktale). Less resources for mitigation and preparedness (before a disaster striking an area to overwhelm local resources), equates to more resources needed for response and recovery during the postdisaster phases of emergency man-agement. Less resources to account for convergence behavior equates to more complexity and complications when there are unexpected volunteers, unexpected forms of miscommunication, and unwanted donations and donors appearing at the doorways and entrances of clinics and hospitals, which is why medical professionals need to design a plan and develop strategies to account for the spontaneous move-ment of human, informational, and logistical resources over space and time. Less strategy equates to more spirit of sickness.

HUMAN RESOURCES

Medical professionals in clinical environments, emergency departments, and hos-pital landscapes will frequently have to improvise during a mass casualty

(MASCAL) situation as local personnel becomes overwhelmed with the unexpected arrival of patients and the overall medical system loses surge capacities and surge capabilities when there is no method of communications to collaborate with stakeholders to coordinate the movement of medical supplies, pharmaceutical products, and transportation vehicles.[30–34] Most organizations have an emergency management plan (EMP) and MASCAL plans; however, many are unaware of how responder communications are complicated by convergence behavior, which is a complex concept that is familiar to many disaster scholars, but it may be less familiar to emergency managers, first responders, and medical professionals who are responsible for daily operations in clinical environments and hospital landscapes.[21–23,25,26]

Several problems emerge from the spontaneous movement of human resources into the domain of disaster response.[21,23] Trained and untrained personnel, as well as well-intentioned volunteers arrive to perform first aid and render services without knowledge of an EMP, much less an incident command system (ICS) that is a principle of emergency management to manage human, informational, and materiel resources, such as an overwhelming amount of donations and donors trying to push supplies and services toward an area over uncertain periods of space and time.[22,24,26,35–39] Therefore, medical professionals should account for convergence behavior to disrupt responder communications in disaster, especially during a MASCAL situation. This concept was discussed by the National Academies of Science to explain how resources spontaneously converge into a disaster-struck area; then there is bifurcation of insiders and outsiders self-organizing, which results in some problems with social control.[21]

When disaster scholars and emergency medicine physicians revisited the concept at the turn of the twentieth century to study disaster response operations shortly after 9/11 in New York City (some lost their lives due to several problems with responder communications and social control), they noticed that there were more issues than inadequate radio frequencies, such as the ineffective ICS when the Emergency Operations Center (EOC) located near the Twin Towers was destroyed and several organizations had to improvise.[10,16,21,22,26,40] The police officers reproduced the EOC setup in a new location, but they did not collaborate with the fire department and medical organizations, which resulted in some freelance medical providers going to the site to perform ad hoc triage while volunteers entered the disaster sites and treatment facilities without authorization or credentials.[16,22] This did not result in more injuries to medical providers (as what happened in Oklahoma when debris fell on a nurse who tried to establish an ad hoc triage site too close to a crumbling building), but firefighters who were unable to receive orders to evacuate the collapsing building were killed due to convergence behavior and problems with responder communications and social control.[10,22,40,41] Today, the ICS is more effective; however, a strategic approach to human resources should account for both expected and unexpected volunteers to arrive in the workspaces of clinics, hospitals, and other medical organizations that usually fall into the public and nonprofit sectors of emergency management and responder communications.[10,26,42,43] With this in mind, cognitive dissonance occurs when well-intentioned people provide resources to feel better about themselves and their safe situation as they see others suffer, so medical organizations should create a strategy to collect data, facilitate dialogue, leverage technology, and organize action to receive donations and supplies (ie, make space for storage of supplies and stowing away goods) that will not discourage humanitarians.[9,24,26,44–46]

INFORMATION RESOURCES

To improve responder communications (in disaster medicine), spokespersons are encouraged to use the IDEA Model "for translating risk and crisis messages effectively to nonscientific publics"—a model rooted in experiential learning theory that uses the acronym *IDEA*: (I) internalization, (D) distribution, (E) explanation, and (A) actions to be taken.[13(p68)] Internalization is supposed to motivate people to pay attention to messages from those who express care and compassion, highlight personal impacts, clarify proximity, indicate timeliness, and use exemplars to answer the personal relevance question: "Am I or those I care about affected and how?"[13(p69)] In order for internalization to work effectively, receivers of a message must believe that the source (ie, spokesperson) is both trustworthy and credible, especially if social media is used to collect data, facilitate dialogue, and leverage technology to both explain what is happening and why, as well as what actions to take for safety and survival, which is difficult when some people tend to ignore messages from strangers.[6–9,12–15,18,28,43,47]

The IDEAL Model may be augmented with a framework of spatial analysis to provide thematic maps, which are visualization tools and may be designed as works of art to improve responder communications (in disaster medicine).[13,48–53] The CDC and other medical organizations publish maps to visualize vulnerable populations by using geospatial data and spatial analysis to measure variables taken from different themes associated with social vulnerability, such as socioeconomic status, housing, and transportation issues.[54–57] Thematic maps may also be used to view everything from heat indexes to the location of season and migrant workers exposed to physical hazards and environmental risks.[58,59] There are also ways to simply illustrate a plan for some external and internal spaces surrounding hospital and clinic landscapes, such as a hand-drawn thematic map to share information about a disaster-struck area (**Fig. 1**).

The legend of a thematic map provides reference points where there is danger in a disaster-struck area, as well as locations to signify how human resources (eg, victims, volunteers, etc.) will move from exterior spaces surrounding a workplace into the interior spaces of clinic and hospital environments, as well as the location of other places, such as a hotel, that may be used as an EOC to share information as first responders (eg, police, firefighters, etc.) improvise to collaborate with stakeholders and coordinate resources for response operations. When the Boston Marathon bombings occurred, there was an ad hoc EOC setup in a hotel as municipal and state leaders started to collaborate with federal agencies to enact both a local EMP and the National Incident-Command Management System established by the National Response Framework and various Emergency Support Function annexes, which helps to coordinate resources from various organizations in the private, public, and nonprofit sectors of emergency management.[43,60–63] Verbal communications may be augmented by visual tools to collect data and share information by leveraging technology with collaborative efforts, which was used by media to report about the Austin bombings that occurred in March 2018.[19] Visual tools, such as thematic maps, will help spokespersons using the IDEAL model when they communicate directly with stakeholders and explain to people that they need to take action if they are located someplace where danger is imminent. Although the IDEA Model and thematic maps are not panaceas, social media and spatial analysis may be used with traditional forms of media (eg, spokespersons, print, radio, television, etc.), as well as alert and warning systems (ie, alarms and sirens). Without social media and spatial analysis to verbalize and visualize landscapes and logistical resources, it is more difficult to *show/tell* responders

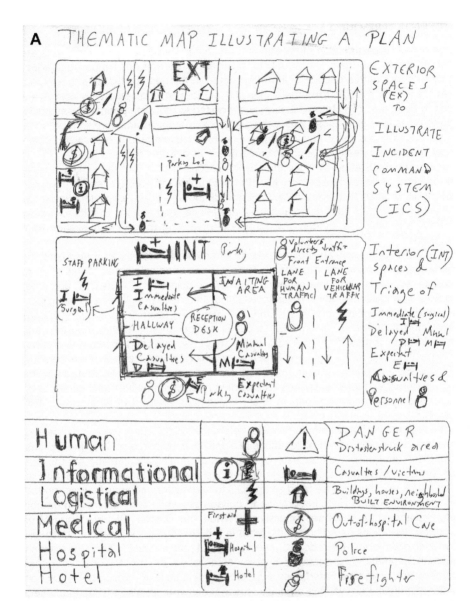

Fig. 1. (*A*) Hand-drawn illustration by primary author to indicate location of resources associated with responder communications in disaster medicine. (*B*) Rendering of hand-drawn thematic map in **fig 1**A.

who/what goes *where/when*. With more destructive disasters, such as catastrophic earthquakes and hurricanes, people need creative forms of improvisation, such as scrounging for cloth and paint and paper and pens to create banners and signs or making a fire to create smoke signals—somewhat akin to castaways pulling together their resources for survival. Within a disaster-struck area, volunteers who are cyclists and runners may be used to establish lines of communications to coordinate logistical resources.

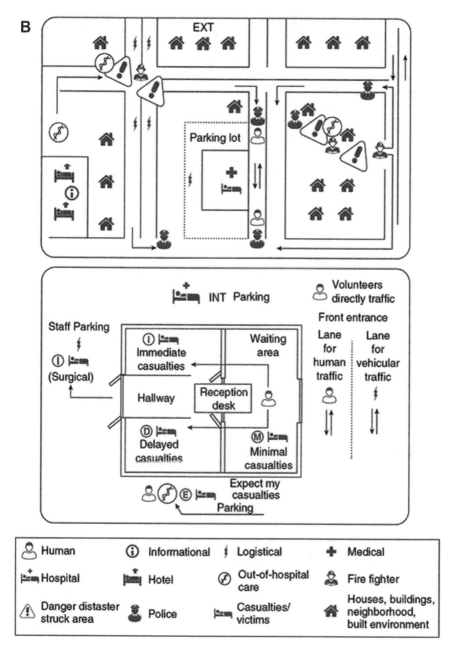

Fig. 1. (*continued*)

LOGISTICAL RESOURCES

The Department of Defense (DOD) uses joint logistics to supply and sustain troops, as well as humanitarian interventions in different places throughout the world when the DOD is ordered to provide Defense Support to Civil Authorities (DSCA) operations.[64] There are 10 classes of supply to sustain people. These supplies include everything from subsistence to repair parts and material not supported by the DOD, such as local contracts to acquire goods and services. They may be seen as symbols and viably placed on thematic maps to indicate what supplies are needed (**Fig. 2**).

Medical logistics (ie, Class VIII) may often be transported by military vehicles that are managed by the National Guard at the state levels of emergency management (ie, Title 32) or part of DSCA operations during a federal response (ie, Title 10).[64] This is important for medical professionals who need to request supplies for surge capacities and surge capabilities, especially when there is an MASCAL situation that overwhelms the limited supply of resources transported to hospitals and clinics.[34,44,65]

Classes, Subclasses of Supply, and Common-User Logistics Suitability

Class	Symbols	Subclass	Common-User Logistics (CUL) Capability
I. Subsistence: Food		A - Nonperishable dehydrated subsistence that requires organized dining facilities C - Combat rations includes meals, ready to eat that require no organized dining facility; used in combat and in-flight environments. Includes gratuitous health and welfare items R - Refrigerated subsistence S - Non-refrigerated subsistence (less other subclasses) W- Water	Fully suited to CUL
II. General Support Items: Clothing, individual equipment, tentage, organizational tool sets and tool kits, hand tools, material, administrative, and housekeeping supplies		A - Air B - Ground support material E - General supplies F - Clothing and textiles G - Electronics M - Weapons T - Industrial supplies (eg, bearings, block and tackle, cable, chain, wire, rope, screws, bolts, studs, steel rods, plates, and bars)	Limited CUL suitability
III. Petroleum, Oils, Lubricants (POL): Petroleum (including packaged items), fuels, lubricants, hydraulic and insulating oils, preservatives, liquids and compressed gasses, coolants, deicing, and antifreeze compounds, plus components and additives of such products, including coal		A - Air W- Ground (surface) P - Packaged POL	Excellent CUL candidate (with some limitations)
IV. Construction/Barrier: Materials that support fortification, obstacle and barrier construction, and construction material for base development and general engineering		A - Construction B - Barrier materials	Fully suited for CUL
V. Ammunition: Ammunition of all types (including chemical, radiological, and special weapons), bombs, explosives, mines, fuses, detonators, pyrotechnics, missiles, rockets, propellants, and other associated items		A - Air W - Ground	Limited, primarily to small arms, selected larger munitions

Fig. 2. Classes of supply taken from DOD publication about joint logistics. (*From* Chairman of the Joint Chiefs of Staff (CJCS.) *Joint Publication 4-0 Joint Logistics.*; 4 February 2019.Available at: https://fas.org/irp/doddir/dod/jp4_0.pdf.)

Responders should inventory their supply chains and try to design thematic maps to indicate how they will transport casualties during an MASCAL situation (see **Fig. 1**). Symbols from Joint Logistics may be drawn on a thematic map to help medical organizations plan resupply when they know military vehicles will be transporting various types of supply material. They may be designed to show where logistical resources will be placed inside the interior spaces of hospitals and clinics, such as a designated area to store essential supplies (eg, fuel for power generators or Class III and Class VII) and stow away personal belongings (ie, Class VI). This type of inventory requires responders to collaborate with stakeholders, such as volunteers, to coordinate the movement of logistical resources into designated spaces that may be part of an EMP or improvised to expand surge capacity and capability during an MASCAL situation.

When large-scale disasters occur, logistical resources and MASCAL situations go hand-in-hand with the movement of human resources and sharing situational reports via an incident command system, especially to those hospitals and clinics that already had limited resources to serve vulnerable populations, such as the extremely young and the extremely old, as well as others with limited socioeconomic, housing, and transportation resources to prepare for and respond to disasters, so humanitarian interventions from private, public, and nonprofit organizations should be coordinated with DOD Joint Logistics to improve responder communications (in disaster medicine).[34,38,44,57,64–70]

SUMMARY

This article asked a metaphysical question: "Is less more?" From a theoretic perspective, "less is a bore" was the counterpoint to the old adage "less is more." In other words, there were old-school versus new-school paradigms to raise questions about complexity versus simplicity in built environments. So what, right?

The *so what* is that the built environment is frequently where responder communications (in disaster medicine) literally takes place, yet it is easy to forget how convergence behavior (ie, spontaneous movement of human, informational, and logistical resources) takes place in a built environment. There will be (un)equipped, (un)expected, (un)trained, and (un)wanted professionals and volunteers arriving at the scene because people are attracted to disasters. They will use social media and spatial analysis to communicate verbally and visually as dispatchers and first responders try to collaborate with stakeholders. They will need to coordinate the movement of logistical resources over space and time. Ultimately, the goal is to collect data, facilitate dialogue, leverage technology, organize action, and share information to improve responder communications (in disaster medicine).

REFERENCES

1. Poulin R. Graphic design + architecture, a 20th century history: a guide to type, image, symbol, and visual Storytelling in the modern world 2012. Vol 50. Beverly (MA): Rockport Publishers; 2013.
2. Fleming J, Honour H, Pevsner N. Penguin dictionary of architecture and landscape architecture. 5th edition. London: Penguin Books; 1999.
3. Curl JS. Oxford dictionary of architecture and landscape architecture. 2nd edition. New York: Oxford University Press; 2006.
4. Gray S, editor. Architects on architects. 1st edition. New York: McGraw-Hill; 2002.

5. Venturi R, Brown DS, Izenour S. Learning from Las Vegas: the forgotten symbolism of architectural form. Cambridge (MA): MIT Press; 1972.

6. Wukich C. Preparing for disaster: social media use for household, organizational, and community preparedness. Risk Hazards Crisis Public Policy 2018;(9999): 9999. https://doi.org/10.1002/rhc3.12161.

7. Bennett D. Emergency preparedness collaboration on Twitter. J Emerg Manag 2018;16(3):191.

8. Wukich C. Social media use in emergency management. J Emerg Manag 2015; 13(4):281.

9. Bennett DM. How do emergency managers use social media platforms? J Emerg Manag 2015;12(3):251.

10. Haddow GD, Bullock JA. Introduction to emergency management. 2nd edition. Burlington (MA): Butterworth-Heinemann Homeland Security Series; 2008.

11. Haddow GD, Haddow KS. Application of communications principles to all four phases of emergency management. Disaster Commun a Chang Media World 2014;93–119. https://doi.org/10.1016/b978-0-12-407868-0.00006-9.

12. Black DR, Dietz JE, Stirratt AA, et al. Do social media have a place in public health emergency response? J Emerg Manag 2015;13(3):217.

13. Sellnow DD, Sellnow TL. The IDEA model for effective instructional risk and crisis communication by emergency managers and other key spokespersons. J Emerg Manag 2019;17(1):67.

14. Siskey A, Islam T. Social media best practices in emergency management. J Emerg Manag 2016;14(2):113.

15. Stern E. Unpacking and Exploring the Relationship between Crisis Management and Social Media in the Era of 'Smart Devices.' Homel Secur Aff. 2017;13(June):article 4. Available at: https://www.hsaj.org/articles/13986.

16. Kendra J, Wachtendorf T. Improvisation, Creativity, and the Art of Emergency Management. In: Durmaz H, Sevinc B, Yayla AS, et al, editors. Understanding and Responding to Terrorism. Fairfax, VA: IOS Press; 2007. p. 324–35.

17. Haddow GD, Haddow KS. Principles of a successful communications strategy. Disaster Commun a Chang Media World 2014;71–92. https://doi.org/10.1016/b978-0-12-407868-0.00005-7.

18. Sutton J, Gibson CB, Spiro ES, et al. What it takes to get passed on: Message content, style, and structure as predictors of retransmission in the Boston Marathon Bombing response. PLoS One 2015;10(8):1–20.

19. Plohetski T. "I still want to know why": one year later, how the Austin bomber was stopped. Austin (TX): KVUE/Austin American-Statesmen; 2019. Available at: https://www.kvue.com/article/news/local/austin-bomber/i-still-want-to-know-why-one-year-later-how-the-austin-bomber-was-stopped/269-a22f0413-ee9c-4020-84f8-64e224895e6c.

20. Murchison SB. Uses of GIS for Homeland Security and Emergency Management for Higher Education Institutions. New Dir Institutional Res 2010;(146):75–86.

21. Auf der Heide E. Convergence behavior in disasters. Ann Emerg Med 2003; 41(4):463–6.

22. Cone DC, Weir SD, Bogucki S. Convergent volunteerism. Ann Emerg Med 2003; 42(6):847.

23. Fritz CE, Mathewson JH. Convergence Behavior as a Problem with Social Control The Rio Grande Flood: Committee on Disaster Studies Academy of Sciences- National Research Council. Washington, DC; 1956. Availabe at: https://archive.org/details/convergencebehav00fritrich.

24. Nelan MM, Wachtendorf T, Penta S. Agility in disaster relief: a social construction approach. Risk Hazards Crisis Public Policy 2018;9(2):132–50.

25. Alexander D, Barton AH, Boin A, et al. What Is a Disaster? New Answers to Old Questions (Vols. I-II). In: Perry RW, Quarantelli EL, editors. Bloomington: Xlibris; 2005. p. 1–442.

26. Waugh WL. Living with hazards, dealing with disasters: an introduction to emergency management. Armonk (NY): M. E. Sharpe; 2000.

27. Schroeder K. Keep it simple, stupid. Disaster Recover J 2009;22(4):24–5. Available at: https://www.drj.com/journal/fall-2009-volume-22-number-4/keep-it-simple-stupid.html.

28. Bean H, Liu BF, Madden S, et al. Disaster Warnings in Your Pocket: How Audiences Interpret Mobile Alerts for an Unfamiliar Hazard. J Contingencies Cris Manag 2016;24(3):136–47.

29. Cleary T (tranlator). The illustrated art of war: by Sun Tzu. 1st edition. Boston (MA): Shambhala Publications; 1998.

30. Willems A, Waxman B, Bacon AK, et al. Interprofessional non-technical skills for surgeons in disaster response: a literature review. J Interprof Care 2013;27(5): 380–6.

31. Oliver J. Creativity as openness: improvising health and care "situations." Health Care Anal 2009;17(4):318–30.

32. Haidet P. Jazz and the "art" of medicine: improvisation in the medical encounter. Ann Fam Med 2007;5(2):164–9.

33. da Graça Batista M, Clegg S, Cunha MP, et al. Improvising prescription: evidence from the emergency room. Br J Manag 2016;27(2):406–25.

34. Runkle JD, Brock-Martin A, Karmaus W, et al. Secondary surge capacity: a framework for understanding long-term access to primary care for medically vulnerable populations in disaster recovery. Am J Public Health 2012;102(12): 24–33.

35. Haddow G. Communications: the critical function. Responding to Catastrophic Events 2016;139–57. https://doi.org/10.1057/9781137336439_8.

36. Reddy MC, Paul SA, Abraham J, et al. Challenges to effective crisis management: Using information and communication technologies to coordinate emergency medical services and emergency department teams. Int J Med Inform 2009;78(4):259–69.

37. Ramasamy A, Midwinter M, Mahoney P, et al. Learning the lessons from conflict: pre-hospital cervical spine stabilisation following ballistic neck trauma. Injury 2009;40(12):1342–5.

38. Rimstad R, Njå O, Rake EL, et al. Incident Command and Information Flows in a Large-Scale Emergency Operation. J Contingencies Cris Manag 2014;22(1): 29–38.

39. Butler FK, Hagmann JH, Richards DT. Tactical management of urban warfare casualties in special operations. Mil Med 2018;165(suppl_1):1–48.

40. Nicholson WC. Emergency response and emergency management law. 1st edition. Springfield (IL): Charles C Thomas; 2003.

41. Erickson PA. Emergency response planning: for corporate and municipal managers. 2nd edition. Burlington (MA): Butterworth-Heinemann; 2006.

42. Pynes JE. Human resources management for public and nonprofit organizations: a strategic approach (Third Edition). 3rd edition. San Francisco (CA): ossey-Bass; 2009.

43. Haddow GD, Haddow KS. Disaster communications in a changing media world: second edition. 2nd edition. Waltham (MA): Butterworth-Heinemann [Adobe Digital Edition]; 2014. https://doi.org/10.1016/C2012-0-06592-1.

44. Safeer M, Anbuudayasankar SP, Balkumar K, et al. Analyzing transportation and distribution in emergency humanitarian logistics. Procedia Eng 2014;97:2248–58.

45. Roman J. Hurricane maria: a preventable humanitarian and health care crisis unveiling the puerto rican dilemma. Ann Am Thorac Soc 2018;15(3):293–5.

46. Waters RD, Tindall NTJ. Exploring the Impact of American News Coverage on Crisis Fundraising: Using Media Theory to Explicate a New Model of Fundraising Communication. J Nonprofit Public Sect Mark 2011;23(1):20–40.

47. Merchant RM, Elmer S, Lurie N. Integrating social media into emergency-preparedness efforts. N Engl J Med 2011;365(4):289–91.

48. Steinitz C. A framework for theory applicable to the education of landscape architects (and other environmental design professionals). Landsc J 1990;9(2): 136–43.

49. Steinitz C. On complexity and scale and the need for spatial analysis. ArcNews 2011. Available at: https://www.esri.com/news/arcnews/spring11articles/on-scale-and-complexity-and-the-need-for-spatial-analysis.html.

50. Wood D. The power of maps. New York: The Guilford Press; 1992.

51. Powell K. Making sense of place: mapping as a multisensory research method. Qual Inq 2010;16(7):539–55.

52. Carroll LN, Au AP, Detwiler LT, et al. Visualization and analytics tools for infectious disease epidemiology: a systematic review. J Biomed Inform 2014;51:287–98.

53. Goodchild MF, Bruzewicz AJ, Cutter SL, et al. Successful response starts with a map: improving geospatial Support for disaster management. Washington, DC: National Academies Press; 2006.

54. Flanagan BE, Hallisey EJ, Adams E, et al. Measuring community vulnerability to natural and anthropogenic hazards: the Centers for Disease Control and Prevention's Social Vulnerability Index. J Environ Health 2018;80(10):34–7.

55. Tate E. Social vulnerability index. Ann Assoc Am Geogr 2013;103(3):526–43.

56. Center for Disease control and prevention (CDC)'s agency for Toxic Substances and Disease Registry (ATSDR). SVI 2016 Documentation - 1/24/2018 2018. Available at: https://svi.cdc.gov/Documents/FactSheet/SVIFactSheet.pdf. Accessed March 15, 2019.

57. Ramisetty-Mikler S, Mikler AR, O'Neill M, et al. Conceptual framework and quantification of population vulnerability for effective emergency response planning. J Emerg Manag 2015;13(3):227.

58. Méndez-Lázaro P, Muller-Karger FE, Otis D, et al. A heat vulnerability index to improve urban public health management in San Juan, Puerto Rico. Int J Biometeorol 2018;62(5):709–22.

59. Montz BE, Allen TR, Monitz GI. Systemic trends in disaster vulnerability: migrant and seasonal farm workers in North Carolina. Risk Hazards Crisis Public Policy 2011;2(1):82–98.

60. Cole CM, Howitt AM, Heymann PB. Why was Boston strong? 2014. Cambridge (MA). Available at: https://ash.harvard.edu/files/why_was_boston_strong.pdf. Accessed March 15, 2019.

61. Helman S, Russell J. Long mile home: Boston under attack, the city's courageous recovery, and the epic hunt for justice. New York: Penguin Group; 2014.

62. Sherman C, Wedge S. Boston strong: a city's triumph over tragedy. Lebanon (NH): ForeEdge (University Press of New England); 2015.

63. Sledge D, Thomas HF. From disaster response to community recovery: nongovernmental entities, government, and public health. Am J Public Health 2019; 109(3):437–44.
64. CJCS (Chairman of the Joint Staff). Joint Publication 4-0 joint logistics. Department of Defense, 2019.
65. Barbera JA, Macintyre AG. Medical surge capacity and capability. Washington, DC: The National Academies Press; 2010. https://doi.org/10.17226/12798.
66. Hoffman S. Preparing for disaster: protecting the most vulnerable in emergencies case Research paper Series in legal Studies 2008. p. 1491–547. Available at: http://ssrn.com/abstract=1268277CASEWESTERNRESERVEUNIVERSITYhttp:// ssrn.com/abstract=1268277http://www.law.case.edu/ssrn. Accessed March 15, 2019.
67. Wexler B, Smith M-E. Disaster response and people experiencing homelessness: addressing challenges of a population with limited resources. J Emerg Manag 2015;13(3):195.
68. Dolan G, Messen D. Social vulnerability: an emergency managers' planning tool. J Emerg Manag 2013;10(3):161.
69. Bethel JW, Foreman AN, Burke SC. Disaster preparedness among medically vulnerable populations. Am J Prev Med 2011;40(2):139–43.
70. Isralowitz R, Findley P. Emergency preparedness and vulnerable populations: lessons learned for education and training. J Emerg Manag 2018;7(6):29.

Chemical Threat
What Physician Assistants Need to Know

Stephan C. Kesterson, MPAS, PA-C[a],*,
Nathaniel J. Taylor, MPAS, PA-C[b],*

KEYWORDS

- Chemical warfare agent • Toxic industrial chemicals • Cyanide • Nerve agent
- Blister agent • Pulmonary agent

KEY POINTS

- Chemical warfare agents are designed to injure, incapacitate, or kill their intended targets, classified by their physiochemical properties and physiologic effects to health.
- Industrial chemicals have the potential to be used for nefarious intent, although accidental release also poses significant risks to populations and local communities.
- Recognition of various chemical toxicants by clinicians may facilitate early diagnosis and medical management for exposed individuals.

INTRODUCTION
Background

On January 23, 1993, the world made a magnificent commitment to stop the stockpiling and production of chemical warfare agents by signing the Chemical Weapons Convention. Every nation, with the exception of Israel (signed, not ratified), Egypt, South Sudan, and North Korea, participated in this momentous act of global cooperation. Therefore, chemical weapons should be nonexistent in every other nation with the exception of the research of countermeasures. On July 23, 2012, the Syrian Foreign Ministry spokesperson publicly confirmed that Syria was in possession of chemical weapons and that they would not be used except to respond to external aggression. No more than 5 months later, the first reports of the Assad regime's use of chemical weapons against the Syrian people were reported. Since 2013, there have been 85 confirmed chemical weapons attacks in Syria and most have been connected to the Syrian government.[1]

Disclosures: None.
[a] Expeditionary Medical Decontamination Team, 2501 Capehart Road, Omaha, NE 68133, USA;
[b] Weapons of Mass Destruction Team, 5636 East McDowell Road Building M5203, Phoenix, AZ 85008, USA
* Corresponding authors.
E-mail addresses: SCKESTERSONPA@GMAIL.COM (S.C.K.); NJTAYLORPA@GMAIL.COM (N.J.T.)

Physician Assist Clin 4 (2019) 701–713
https://doi.org/10.1016/j.cpha.2019.06.001
2405-7991/19/© 2019 Elsevier Inc. All rights reserved.

physicianassistant.theclinics.com

Not being limited to the Eastern world, on September 5, 2018, Theresa May publicly affirmed that Russian operatives used nerve agents to attack a former spy and his daughter in Salisbury, United Kingdom. Further raising the stakes, this was the first leader within the Western world to publicly use the term Novichok, affirming a previously unconfirmed class of Russian-designed nerve agent of political and medical significance. Subsequently, an unconnected woman, Dawn Sturgess, was killed by the same substance found in the discarded cosmetic bottle used for the original attack, which she later received as a gift. All of these cases are indications that the threat from chemical warfare agents, although rare, is real. Furthermore, with the introduction of a new generation of chemical agents, every book on the matter is instantly outdated.

As such, the use of chemical agents, whether intentional or incidental, weaponized or industrialized, presents significant challenges to clinicians involved in conventional warfare, terrorist events, natural disasters, and/or major accidents. It is imperative that clinicians maintain awareness of localized vulnerabilities/threats as well as symptom recognition and treatment of any suspected contaminated casualty. Although there is not enough space in this article to provide an exhaustive explanation of these threats, prehospital and response actions, patient decontamination, timely exposure history, and the nuances of treatment for each, this article briefly covers a few agents by class, general approach considerations, and key-point take-home facts on treatments to provide clinicians with actions to move through the initial response to a variety of traditional warfare and chemical agents. In addition, the newly revealed Novichok, or fourth-generation agents, are discussed in order to provide clinicians with a general fluency with which to establish a treatment approach.

Chemical Agents Designed for Warfare and Terrorism

Cyanides
Cyanide is a dual-use agent, meaning it is both a toxic industrial chemical as well as a substance with utility that can be weaponized to incapacitate or kill people. The use of cyanides in large quantities for industrial purposes makes it a readily available substance for those who would use it with nefarious intent. Cyanide is a term that references the anion CN^- or to its acidic form HCN. Cyanogen has a chemical form (C_2N_2), but the term additionally refers to substances that form cyanide once metabolized.[2] Cyanides are present in salt form for industrial use, within nitriles, in plastics, and in many common food sources. In high enough concentrations, cyanides can be deadly by prohibiting intracellular oxygen use through binding to the iron in cytochrome a_3 in the mitochondria of cells.[3]

In less than a minute of exposure to a lethal dose of cyanide, hyperpnea sets in with convulsions followed by termination of respirations within 2 to 3 minutes, followed by death at approximately 6 to 8 minutes after exposure.[2] Despite the similar sounds of the words cyanide and cyanosis, cyanide exposure does not necessarily result in cyanotic appearance of skin. The inability of the cells of the body to use oxygen results in a significant increase in the redness of the venous blood within the body. This inability to use oxygen precludes the preponderance of deoxygenated hemoglobin necessary to produce cyanosis.

Cyanide is one of the few hazardous chemicals for which there are specific antidotes. There are 2 separate treatment paradigms that can be embarked on in addition to traditional supportive care associated with patient management and resuscitation of any toxic substance. The first and older treatment approach consists of a 3-drug treatment kit consisting of amyl nitrite (ampules for inhalation), sodium nitrite (intravenous [IV]), and sodium thiosulfate (IV). The function of the amyl nitrate and sodium nitrate is to initiate methemoglobinemia in approximately 15% of the blood. The goal of this therapy is to exploit the preferential binding of cyanide to methemoglobin rather than cytochrome a_3. Methemoglobinemia is a degraded state for blood to transport oxygen. However, the ability of methemoglobin to pull cyanide and allow cellular respiration to resume is lifesaving. The sodium thiosulfate donates the required sulfur to the natural enzymatic processes that convert cyanide into a renally excretable product.[4] The other treatment approach is much more simple (and more expensive) in the form of hydroxocobalamin. Combined with cyanide, hydroxocobalamin forms the compound cyanocobalamin, which is more commonly known as vitamin B_{12}. Although the performance of these two treatment approaches has not been evaluated in conjunction with one another, sodium thiosulfate independently may be used with hydroxocobalamin as a dual-therapy option. Associated symptoms and treatment of cyanide exposure are reiterated in **Table 1**.[2,5]

Nerve Agents

In the 1930s, German scientists developed nerve agents while creating an organophosphate insecticide. This was significant to the extent that it caught the attention of the Nazi-controlled government. These agents were volatile and lacked persistence in nature. Once armed with the concept, the United Kingdom developed a persistent weaponized organophosphate for war named VX, which was later stolen by the Russians, modified, and renamed Russian VX or RVX. Until January of 2018, the German nerve agents, or G-series agents, and VX-style agents (V-series agents) were the only true nerve agents publicly recognized by Western governments. Subsequently, a newer generation of nerve agents named "Novichocks", "fourth-generation agents", or "A-series agents" have been identified as a chemical weapon threat. They are more persistent than other nerve agents and are at least as toxic as VX. Although fourth-generation agents share similar characteristics with other nerve agents, fourth-generation agents also pose several unique challenges in terms of toxicity, detection, persistence, and potential for delayed onset of symptoms.[6]

Organophosphates are essentially select esters of phosphoric acid that are liquids at room temperature and function by binding acetylcholinesterase (AChE). At neuromuscular junctions, AChE serves to catalyze the neurotransmitter acetylcholine and other choline-based neurotransmitters. The inhibition of cholinesterase blocks the activity of AChE and causes an accumulation of acetylcholine at cholinergic receptors, resulting in persistent receptor stimulation.[4] These inhibitors all have the potential to permanently bind AChE in a process called aging if not appropriately treated. The aging half-life is particular to the nerve agent being used but of special note is soman, which has an aging half-life of 2-minutes. Signs and symptoms of these exposures are cholinergic and peripherally affect muscarinic and nicotinic sites. The cholinergic crisis is often communicated in acronyms for each. Muscarinic signs and symptoms are DUMBELS (diarrhea, urination, miosis, bradycardia, bronchorrhea, bronchospasm, emesis, lacrimation, salivation, secretion, and sweating). Of particular note, the so-called killer Bs of bradycardia, bronchorrhea, and bronchospasm are the mechanism of death in most affected patients. Also, miosis may not be present in patients with isolated dermal exposure as opposed to vapor exposure to the eyes and mucosal tissues of the face. The nicotinic signs and symptoms form the acronym MTWHF (mydriasis, tachycardia, weakness, hypertension, hyperglycemia, and fasciculations) in a days of the week format. Centrally, these patients develop confusion, convulsions, and coma.[4]

The approach recommendations provided by the Department of Health and Human Services does not differ much in consideration across the G-series, V-series, and A-series agents. Removal of clothing and appropriate decontamination of skin with soap and water are necessary measures before hospital management of these patients. However,

Table 1
Cyanide toxicant

Route of Exposure	Symptoms	Medical Management/ Treatment
Inhalation, skin/eye contact, ingestion	Symptoms are dose dependent and may progress if exposure continues. Symptoms associated with lower-concentration exposure may occur within minutes. These symptoms include hyperpnea/dyspnea, anxiety, tachycardia, chest pain, diaphoresis, confusion/ lethargy, nausea/vomiting, and headache. Severe exposure may cause symptoms within seconds and lead to rapid respiratory failure, convulsions, and dysrhythmias/asystole within minutes	Prehospital care should include disrobing and decontaminating any patient reporting irritant complaints following any suspected exposure. In any case of ingestion, no decontamination is necessary, although gavage and activated charcoal are recommended. Any vomitus should be collected to minimize secondary contamination. Execute resuscitation efforts on initial examination, including establishing an airway, administering 100% oxygen, and intubating/ providing mechanical respiratory support if necessary. Reassess circulatory status and administer IV crystalloids/ vasopressors if needed. Also correct any metabolic acidosis with IV sodium bicarbonate. For seizure control, administer benzodiazepine. For patients with severe symptoms, use antidotal therapy with either Cyanokit or the 2-step process amyl nitrite pearls/sodium nitrite infusion. Monitor for overproduction of methemoglobin and use caution for patients with smoke inhalation if amyl nitrite pearls are administered. Also monitor for hypotension if amyl nitrite is administered. Most, if not all, patients need continuous observation and ICU admission

Abbreviation: ICU, intensive care unit.

Data from Banks, D. E., & Borden Institute (U.S.). (2014). Medical management of chemical casualties handbook (Fifth edition. ed.). Fort Sam Houston, Texas: Borden Institute, U.S. Army Medical Department Center and School and Agency for Toxic Substances & Disease Registry. Medical Management for Cyanide. https://www.atsdr.cdc.gov/substances/toxsubstance.asp?toxid=19. Accessed January 19, 2019.

all of the classic treatment drugs that can be given for these patients intravenously (anticholinergics, oximes, benzodiazepines) can also be administered intramuscularly by hazmat first responders in a prehospital setting before full decontamination. Given the cholinergic "wet" types of symptoms discussed earlier, the mainstay of managing this type of crisis is naturally anticholinergic drugs, specifically atropine, which is the US Food and Drug Administration (FDA)–approved anticholinergic for organophosphate poisoning. However, scopolamine has been suggested as another effective medication. These medications should be titrated to bronchorrhea and bradycardia symptoms and not with the intent of reversing the entire cholinergic syndrome because signs such as miosis may not resolve for weeks. It is important not to underestimate the amount of atropine required to manage a casualty of a weaponized nerve agent. Multiple doses should be on hand throughout the treatment of the patient. In addition, pralidoxime is an oxime that is approved to remove and reactivate organophosphate-bound AChE before aging. It has varying efficacy depending on which agent the patient was exposed to, but it is the only commercially available oxime in the United States that is FDA approved for this purpose and should be used empirically for patients showing classic organophosphate poisoning symptoms with a known organophosphate exposure or an unknown cause. Atropine and pralidoxime work synergistically in the management of these patients. Associated convulsions from organophosphate exposure can be managed with midazolam as the drug of choice, lorazepam, or classically with diazepam.[7] Short-acting beta-agonists and ipratropium bromide may also be efficacious for nerve agent–related respiratory decompensation. Positive pressure or mechanical ventilation may also be required. Although all of these agents may result in death despite treatment, the newer the class of agent used for an attack, the greater the lethality. Toxicant exposure, symptoms, and treatment are consolidated in **Table 2**.[2]

Chemicals Designed for Industrial Use (Toxic Industrial Chemicals)

As safeguards limit access to traditional and newer sophisticated warfare agents, industrial chemicals pose additional threats based on easier accessibility and prevalence, volume, lower production costs, and footprint of impact. In 2007, Congress enacted regulatory oversight using risk and vulnerability assessments to identify high-risk chemical facilities, leading to the development of the Chemical Facilities Anti-terrorism Standards, reauthorized and amended through the Protecting and Securing Chemical Facilities from Terrorist Attacks Act in 2014.[8] **Table 3** identifies a sample of the many common industrial chemicals that are manufactured, stored, and distributed. An extensive list of these chemicals of interest can be found in the Code of Federal Regulations (CFR) 27 Part 6.[9,10] Health effects from industrial chemical exposure depend on many variables, including physical state and stability, method and quantity of release/toxicity, route of entry, and environmental factors.[10] In addition, regulatory agencies such as the Environmental Protection Agency (EPA), as well as other federal entities such as the Centers for Disease Control and Prevention (CDC), Occupational Safety and Health Agency (OSHA), and the National Institutes of Health (NIH), provide lay information and public right to know regarding chemical inventories.

Pulmonary Irritant Choking Agents

Phosgene CG, also known as carbonyl dichloride or carbonic dichloride ($COCl_2/CCl_2O$), is an industrial chemical of interest given its use as an intermediate in manufacturing processing, primarily released during synthesis of various esters, polymers, and chlorides by heating or burning these solvents and chemicals.[2] Its battlefield introduction during World War I by Germany contributed to an estimated 85% of all chemical deaths.[11,12] Phosgene is a colorless gas with an olfactory description of newly mown

Table 2
Nerve agent toxicant

Route of Exposure	Symptoms	Medical Management/Treatment
Inhalation, Skin/Eye contact	Symptoms are dose dependent, which may progress if exposure continues. Lethal concentrations differ by physical state because nerve agents are volatile and more toxic in vapor form. However, penetration may occur if chemical is occluded without the ability to off-gas, resulting in an increase in lethality. Symptoms can be focal to targeted area exposed with mild exposure, such as miosis, visual disturbances, lacrimation, headache, rhinorrhea, salivation, and dyspnea when inhaled. Symptoms associated with lower concentrations may occur within seconds to minutes. Severe exposure may lead to rapid respiratory failure, bronchorrhea, emesis, muscular fasciculations, convulsions, paralysis, loss of bowel and bladder control, cyanosis, bradycardia, and death within seconds to minutes. Mild to moderate contact exposure can cause focal fasciculations at site of exposure, sweating at exposure site, nausea and vomiting, and lethargy. Symptoms may occur within minutes to hours, and sooner if area is occluded. Severe contact exposure may lead to symptoms similar to those associated with vapor inhalation	Prehospital care should include disrobing and decontaminating any patient who may have contact exposure for trapped vapor hazard concerns. Execute resuscitation efforts on initial examination, including establishing an airway, administering 100% oxygen, and intubating/providing mechanical respiratory support if necessary. Early administration of antidotal therapy may be necessary (atropine and pralidoxime chloride). Albuterol for bronchospasm after antidotal therapy. Consider short-acting beta-agonist such as ipratropium bromide for respiratory decompensation. For seizure control, administer benzodiazepine. Most, if not all, patients need continuous observation and ICU admission

Data from Banks, DE., & Borden Institute (U.S.). (2014). Medical management of chemical casualties handbook (Fifth edition. ed.). Fort Sam Houston, Texas: Borden Institute, U.S. Army Medical Department Center and School.

hay, corn, or grass that can cause acute and chronic lung injury, dose dependent in both peripheral and central airway compartments.[2] The toxicodynamic effects of phosgene target the bronchioles and alveoli by hydrolyzing and forming hydrochloric acid (HCl) leading to cell death and anoxia. Multiple animal and mechanistic studies confirm the unique latent effects of phosgene to these compartments, because respiratory symptom onset may be insidious rather than immediate compared with other inhaled chemical irritants.[2,13] Initial symptoms may include mucosal membrane irritation and inflammation to the eyes and upper airway, which can occur anywhere from 2 to 24 hours after exposure. As noted, any systemic involvement or major symptom manifestation may go unnoticed up to 72 hours. These symptoms may include dyspnea on

Table 3
Toxic industrial chemicals by hazard index

High	Medium	Low
Ammonia (CAS# 7664-41-7)	Acetone cyanohydrin (CAS# 75-86-5)	Allyl isothiocyanate (CAS# 57-06-7)
Arsine (CAS# 7784-42-1)	Acrolein (CAS# 107-02-8)	Arsenic trichloride (CAS# 7784-34-1)
Boron trichloride (CAS# 10294-34-5)	Acrylonitrile (CAS# 107-13-1)	Bromine (CAS# 7726-95-6)
Boron trifluoride (CAS# 7637-07-2)	Allyl alcohol (CAS# 107-18-6)	Bromine chloride (CAS# 13863-41-7)
Carbon disulfide (CAS# 75-15-0)	Allylamine (CAS# 107-11-9)	Bromine pentafluoride (CAS# 7789-30-2)
Chlorine (CAS# 7782-50-5)	Allyl chlorocarbonate (CAS# 2937-50-0)	Bromine trifluoride (CAS# 7787-71-5)
Diborane (CAS# 19287-45-7)	Boron tribromide (CAS# 10294-33-4)	Carbonyl fluoride (CAS# 353-50-4)
Ethylene oxide (CAS# 75-21-8)	Carbon monoxide (CAS# 630-08-0)	Chlorine pentafluoride (CAS# 13637-63-3)
Fluorine (CAS# 7782-41-4)	Carbonyl sulfide (CAS# 463-58-1)	Chlorine trifluoride (CAS# 7790-91-2)
Formaldehyde (CAS# 50-00-0)	Chloroacetone (CAS# 78-95-5)	Chloroacetaldehyde (CAS# 107-20-0)
Hydrogen bromide (CAS# 10035-10-6)	Chloroacetonitrile (CAS# 7790-94-5)	Chloroacetyl chloride (CAS# 79-04-9)
Hydrogen chloride (CAS# 7647-01-0)	Chlorosulfonic acid (CAS# 7790-94-5)	Crotonaldehyde (CAS# 123-73-9)
Hydrogen cyanide (CAS# 74-90-8)	Diketene (CAS# 674-82-8)	Cyanogen chloride (CAS# 506-77-4)
Hydrogen fluoride (CAS# 7664-39-3)	1,2-Dimethylhydrazine (CAS# 540-73-8)	Dimethyl sulfate (CAS# 77-78-1)
Hydrogen sulfide (CAS# 7783-0604)	Ethylene dibromide (CAS# 106-93-4)	Diphenylmethane-4,4'-diisocyanate (CAS# 101-68-8)
Nitric acid, fuming (CAS# 7697-37-2)	Hydrogen selenide (CAS# 7783-07-5)	Ethyl chloroformate (CAS# 541-41-3)
Phosgene (CAS# 75-44-5)	Methanesulfonyl chloride (CAS# 124-63-0)	Ethyl chlorothioformate (CAS# 2941-64-2)
Phosphorus trichloride (CAS# 7719-12-2)	Methyl bromide (CAS# 74-83-9)	Ethyl phosphonothioic dichloride (CAS# 993-43-1)
Sulfur dioxide (CAS# 7446-09-5)	Methyl chloroformate (CAS# 79-22-1)	Ethyl phosphonic dichloride (CAS# 1066-50-8)
Sulfuric acid (CAS# 7664-93-9)	Methyl chlorosilane (CAS# 993-00-0)	Ethyleneimine (CAS# 151-56-4)
Tungsten hexafluoride (CAS# 7783-82-6)	Methyl hydrazine (CAS# 60-34-4)	Hexachlorocyclopentadiene (CAS# 77-47-4)

(continued on next page)

Table 3
(continued)

High	Medium	Low
	Methyl isocyanate (CAS# 624-83-9)	Hydrogen iodide (CAS# 10034-85-2)
	Methyl mercaptan (CAS# 74-93-1)	Iron pentacarbonyl (CAS# 13463-40-6)
	Nitrogen dioxide (CAS# 10102-44-0)	Isobutyl chloroformate (CAS# 543-27-1)
	Phosphine (CAS# 7803-51-2)	Isopropyl chloroformate (CAS# 108-23-6)
	Phosphorus oxychloride (CAS# 10025-87-3)	Isopropyl isocyanate (CAS# 1795-48-8)
	Phosphorus pentafluoride (CAS# 7647-19-0)	n-Butyl chloroformate (CAS# 592-34-7)
	Selenium hexafluoride (CAS# 7783-79-1)	n-Butyl isocyanate (CAS# 111-36-4)
	Silicon tetrafluoride (CAS# 7783-61-1)	Nitric oxide (CAS# 10102-43-9)
	Stibine (CAS# 7803-52-3)	n-Propyl chloroformate (CAS# 109-61-5)
	Sulfur trioxide (CAS# 7446-11-9)	Parathion (CAS#: 56-38-2)
	Sulfuryl chloride (CAS# 7791-25-5)	Perchloromethyl mercaptan (CAS# 594-42-3)
	Sulfuryl fluoride (CAS# 2699-79-8)	sec-Butyl chloroformate (CAS# 17462-58-7)
	Tellurium hexafluoride (CAS# 7783-80-4)	tert-Butyl isocyanate (CAS# 1609-86-5)
	n-Octyl mercaptan (CAS# 111-88-6)	Tetraethyl lead (CAS# 78-00-2)
	Titanium tetrachloride (CAS# 7550-45-0)	Tetraethyl pyrophosphate (CAS# 107-49-3)
	Trichloroacetyl chloride (CAS# 76-02-8)	Tetramethyl lead (CAS# 75-74-1)
	Trifluoroacetyl chloride (CAS# 354-32-5)	Toluene 2.4-diisocyanate (CAS# 584-84-9)
		Toluene 2.6-diisocyanate (CAS# 91-08-7)

Abbreviation: CAS, Chemical Abstracts Service.

exertion, dyspnea at rest, dysphonia, dysphagia, as well as the killer Bs noted with organophosphates (bronchorrhea, bradycardia, and bronchospasm). Observation is recommended 48 to 72 hours in all patients with phosgene exposure, especially those who may develop impending respiratory failure.[14] Additional information regarding phosgene exposure symptoms and treatment can be seen in **Table 4**.[2,14]

Like phosgene, chlorine (Cl_2) was used in warfare during World War I, becoming the first chemical agent used effectively in battle.[2] Its use in modern society is ubiquitous, in both industrial and consumer applications. Chlorine has a pungent odor and can be seen as a yellow or green haze with large off-gas plumes. Toxic inhalation of chlorine has an immediate effect on the upper respiratory system, affecting both the peripheral and central compartments of the lungs. The proposed mechanism associated with chlorine inhalation is the formation of hydrochloric and hypochlorous acid through hydration in the central compartment, injuring respiratory mucosa.[15] Initial symptoms with chlorine inhalation are similar to those from exposure to phosgene, although symptoms are immediate rather than latent. Treatment of suspected inhaled chlorine exposure can be seen in **Table 4**.[2]

Anhydrous ammonia (NH_3) is another chemical of interest commonly found in rural areas, where roughly 80% is manufactured for use in fertilizer, although it is prevalent in other industrial processes and common household cleaners.[16] Its alkaline properties are focal to the sites of direct contact, similar to both phosgene and chloride (skin, inhalation, ingestion). Ammonia dissolves into ammonium hydroxide, a weak base, on contact with mucosa, which can lead to corrosion and necrosis of tissue. In vapor form, ammonia is a colorless gas that has an overwhelming pungent odor detected with lower concentrations; however, olfactory fatigue can occur.[17] Symptoms and medical management for ammonia are similar to those for phosgene and chlorine with supportive care.[2,17]

Table 4 Pulmonary agent toxicant		
Route of Exposure	**Symptoms**	**Medical Management/Treatment**
Inhalation	Patient may present with eye irritation, rhinorrhea, and pharyngitis leading up to dyspnea upon exertion with moderate concentrated exposures. Dyspnea at rest may indicate heavy concentration exposure. Patients with pulmonary complaints can also have associated frothy secretions and coughing/wheezing, indicating early edema and potential acute respiratory distress. Additional symptoms may include dysphonia/dysphagia as well as laryngospasms and bronchospasms.	Prehospital care should include disrobing and decontaminating any patient reporting irritant complaints following any suspected exposure. Execute resuscitation efforts upon initial examination. Establish airway and administer oxygen. Intubate if necessary. Re-assess circulatory status often for hypotension induced by pulmonary edema. Administer theophylline or beta adrenergic bronchodilators for bronchospasms. For any supplemental positive pressure support or rapid IV colloid/crystalloid administration, seek additional guidance and admit to ICU.

Data from Banks, DE., & Borden Institute (U.S.). (2014). Medical management of chemical casualties handbook (Fifth edition. ed.). Fort Sam Houston, Texas: Borden Institute, U.S. Army Medical Department Center and School and Agency for Toxic Substances & Disease Registry. Medical Management Guidelines for Ammonia. https://www.atsdr.cdc.gov/MHMI/mmg126.pdf. Accessed March 26, 2019.

Blister Vesicant Agents

Introduced during the 1800s, sulfur mustard (H, HD) became a known chemical during World War I, causing more nonlethal casualties than any other agent designed for warfare use.[2] In modern conflicts, such as those between Iraq and Iran during the 1980s,

Table 5 Sulfur mustard toxicant		
Route of Exposure	Symptoms	Medical Management/Treatment
Skin contact	Patients may present with a delayed presentation of erythema of the skin, similar to a sunburn, experiencing burning, pruritus, and pain. Intertriginous areas may be more susceptible given thinner skin and increased humidity. Vesicular eruption may occur, with coalescent features that eventually morph to bullae. Bullae fill with a clear fluid that eventually turns straw color and yellow. As noted, blister fluid does not contain mustard toxicant. In severe exposure cases, necrosis may occur. Ophthalmic symptoms may cause irritation to eyes	Prehospital care should include disrobing and decontaminating any patient reporting dermal complaints following an event. For erythema, calamine or other soothing lotion (0.25% camphor and menthol) should be provided for any irritation. Vesicular rashes should be left intact, although for larger bullae, unroofing or aspiration can be performed. Denuded areas should be irrigated every 6–8 h with topical antibiotic such as silver sulfadiazine or mafenide acetate at least 1–2 mm thickness applied to affected area. Systemic analgesics and antipruritics as needed for pain and itching. Consider hospitalization and wound clinic consult for additional management. For ophthalmic symptoms, flushing of eyes with ophthalmic solutions should be done generously. Use of homatropine ointment helps prevent further synechiae and Vaseline ointment should be applied to prevent further scarring. In addition, conservative measures, such as sunglass use, should be recommended to minimize photophobia. Consult with ophthalmology for additional recommendations
Inhalation	Symptoms of sore throat, hoarseness, and dyspnea can be expected with concentrated vapor exposure. Patients may experience secondary bacterial symptoms after 72 h, such as fever, leukocytosis, and productive cough, although this can be seen within 24 h. In addition, for heavier systemic exposure, mild cholinergic symptoms as well as bone marrow suppression may occur	Intubate if necessary. Antibiotics for suspected bacterial infection. For any supplemental positive pressure support or rapid IV colloid/crystalloid administration, seek additional guidance and admit to ICU

Data from Banks, DE., & Borden Institute (U.S.). (2014). Medical management of chemical casualties handbook (Fifth edition. ed.). Fort Sam Houston, Texas: Borden Institute, U.S. Army Medical Department Center and School.

the use of mustard gas necessitates continued treatment for nearly one-third of nonfatal casualties sustaining cutaneous, ocular, respiratory, and gastrointestinal injuries.[18] The mechanism by which sulfur mustard acts allows it to bind to cellular enzymes and other components, alkylating DNA with subsequent oxidative stress, inflammation, and apoptosis to various tissues and organs.[2] Furthermore, lipophilic properties enhance its effectiveness, similar to other vesicant and nettle-urticant agents; however, immediate symptoms of irritation and pain are not seen with sulfur mustard, which may cause a delay in seeking decontamination.[19] In addition, topical and systemic symptoms may not manifest for hours, dependent on exposure severity as well as physiochemical state during contact. However, because sulfur mustard reacts with tissue and enters the body, clinicians should be aware that blister fluid, tissue, and blood products contain no free mustard, creating zero risk for contamination when encountered.[2] **Table 5** lists symptoms and medical management for suspected exposures.[2]

Lewisite (L), another known vesicant, was also introduced in the early 1900s, although at the end of World War I and not used on the battlefield. Unlike mustard, lewisite burns immediately, causing anyone exposed to seek immediate decontamination.[2] In addition, absorption of lewisite can cause capillary permeability leading to hypovolemic shock and end-organ damage. Management for lewisite is similar to that for mustard, although an antidote (BAL [British Anti-Lewisite]) is available to aid in treatment of skin, ophthalmic, and systemic symptoms.

Phosgene oxime (CX) is an urticant or nettle agent in that it does not create bullae with classic vesicants, but does cause systemic urticaria and wheals on exposure. As with lewisite, the toxicodynamics of phosgene oxime are not fully known. Symptoms are also immediate and extremely painful to the eyes and mucous membranes, leading to early suspicion in the acute setting of systemic pruritus and pain out of proportion. Management for exposure should be supportive with care for any skin lesions.[2]

Note that, with any chemical exposure, consultation with industrial hygienists, toxicologists, as well specialists for vulnerable populations, such as pediatric, immunocompromised, geriatric, and pregnant, is recommended.

SUMMARY

Chemicals are ubiquitous in the communities that clinicians serve and that provide a purpose to our way of life. Ironically, they also create a public health risk. Clinicians

---

Box 1
Recommended reading: United States Department of Health and Human Services guidelines for acute patient care of nerve agents

https://chemm.nlm.nih.gov/nerveagents.htm

https://chemm.nlm.nih.gov/lungagents.htm

https://www.atsdr.cdc.gov/MHMI/mmg176.pdf

https://www.atsdr.cdc.gov/MHMI/mmg172.pdf

https://www.atsdr.cdc.gov/MHMI/mmg126.pdf

https://www.atsdr.cdc.gov/MHMI/mmg165.pdf

https://www.atsdr.cdc.gov/mhmi/mmg163.pdf

https://www.atsdr.cdc.gov/MHMI/mmg167.pdf

must have an understanding of the potential harms associated with chemical contact to appropriately manage the challenges they present, regardless of exposure scale. In addition, preparation and training can help optimize rapid assessment and treatment in the chain of chemical survival; therefore, it is clinicians' responsibility to remain medically steadfast in response to future chemical events (**Box 1**).

REFERENCES

1. Syria: a year on, chemical weapons attacks persist. 2018. Available at: https://www.hrw.org/news/2018/04/04/syria-year-chemical-weapons-attacks-persist.
2. Banks, D. E., Borden Institute (U.S.. Medical management of chemical casualties handbook. 5th edition. Fort Sam Houston (TX): Borden Institute, U.S. Army Medical Department Center and School; 2014.
3. Tuorinsky SD. Medical aspects of chemical warfare. Falls Church (VA): Office of the Surgeon General, U.S. Army; 2008.
4. McFee RB, Leikin JB. Toxico-terrorism : emergency response and clinical approach to chemical, biological, and radiological agents. New York: McGraw-Hill, Health Professions Division; 2008.
5. Agency for Toxic Substances & Disease Registry. Medical Management for Cyanide. Available at: https://www.atsdr.cdc.gov/substances/toxsubstance.asp?toxid=19. Accessed January 19, 2019.
6. U.S. Department of Health & Human Services. Fourth Generation Agents. Available at: https://chemm.nlm.nih.gov/nerveagents/FGA.htm. Accessed February 20, 2019.
7. Reddy SD, Reddy DS. Midazolam as an anticonvulsant antidote for organophosphate intoxication–A pharmacotherapeutic appraisal. Epilepsia 2015;56(6): 813–21. Available at: https://www.ncbi.nlm.nih.gov/pubmed/26032507.
8. United States Department of Homeland Security. Chemical facility Ant-terrorism Standards. Available at: https://www.dhs.gov/cisa/chemical-facility-anti-terrorism-standards. Accessed January 31, 2019.
9. United States Department of Homeland Security. Appendix A: Chemicals of Interest (COI). Available at: https://www.dhs.gov/cisa/appendix-chemicals-interest. Accessed January 31, 2019.
10. United States Department of Labor. Occupational safety and health Administration toxic industrial chemicals Guide. Available at: https://www.osha.gov/SLTC/emergencypreparedness/guides/chemical.html. Accessed March 12, 2019.
11. Fitzgerald GJ. Chemical warfare and medical response during World War I [published correction appears in Am J Public Health. 2008 Jul;98(7):1158]. Am J Public Health 2008;98(4):611–25.
12. Jones E. Terror weapons: The British experience of gas and its treatment in the first world war. War Hist 2014;21(3):355–75.
13. Li W, Pauluhn J. Phosgene-induced acute lung injury (ALI): differences from chlorine-induced ALI and attempts to translate toxicology to clinical medicine. Clin Transl Med 2017;6(1):19.
14. Agency for Toxic Substances & Disease Registry. Medical management for phosgene. Available at: https://www.atsdr.cdc.gov/mmg/mmg.asp?id=1201&tid=182. Accessed February 19, 2019.
15. White CW, Martin JG. Chlorine gas inhalation: human clinical evidence of toxicity and experience in animal models. Proc Am Thorac Soc 2010;7(4):257–63.

16. Agency for Toxic Substances & Disease Registry. Toxicological profile for ammonia. Available at: https://www.atsdr.cdc.gov/toxprofiles/tp126.pdf. Accessed March 26, 2019.
17. Agency for Toxic Substances & Disease Registry. Medical management Guidelines for ammonia. Available at: https://www.atsdr.cdc.gov/MHMI/mmg126.pdf. Accessed March 26, 2019.
18. Nokhodian Z, ZareFarashbandi F, Shoaei P. Mustard gas exposure in Iran-Iraq war - A scientometric study. J Educ Health Promot 2015;4:56.
19. Agency for Toxic Substances & Disease Registry. Medical management for sulfur mustard. Available at: https://www.atsdr.cdc.gov/MHMI/mmg165.pdf. Accessed April 24, 2019.

Radioactive Contaminated Patients

Larry Reeder, RRPT, BS Technology[a],*, Nathaniel J. Taylor, MPAS, PA-C[b]

KEYWORDS

- Radiation • Contamination • Handling • Treatment

KEY POINTS

- What is radiation?
- Handling and treatment of radioactive contaminated patients.
- Clinicians' perspective.
- Event-oriented and patient-oriented medical approach.

INTRODUCTION
Background

February 2019: A hospital in Orlando Florida
I have just been wheeled into my room after a total knee replacement. While getting situated, the aide asked 'What do you do for a living'? My reply is that I am a radiation protection technologist with a nuclear facility. To which the aide replies, "When I hear that a patient has radiation stuff on board I try to stay away."

This article discusses several incidents that have occurred in the previous 20 years and that have led to situations in which personnel with radioactive contamination needed medical treatment (**Box 1**). Radioactive contamination is a scary expression for many, as was shown by the aide helping me after my surgery. However, it should not be. Everyone in the medical field has the knowledge and training to safely treat patients who have radiological contamination.

What is radiation contamination and why are people scared of it? As with most things that are frightening, it is usually caused by a lack of understanding. People cannot feel it, see it, or taste it. They cannot feel, see, or taste germs; however, they know they are there and they use precautions to protect themselves. However, if radioactive material is suspected, then using the proper equipment can detect it, sometimes immediately.

Disclosure: The authors have nothing to disclose.
[a] Duke Energy Florida - NA2B, 15760 W Powerline Street, Crystal River, FL 34428, USA; [b] 91st Weapons of Mass Destruction Team, 5636 E. McDowell Road, M203, Phoenix, AZ 85008, USA
* Corresponding author.
E-mail address: l.reeder55@gmail.com

Box 1
Incidents of radioactive contamination

- April 2010, New Delhi, India: a 35-year-old man is hospitalized after handling radioactive scrap metal. Investigation led to the discovery of an amount of scrap metal containing colbalt-60 (Co-60, a radioactive material used in industrial applications such as sterilization) in the New Delhi industrial district of Mayapuri. The man later died of his injuries, and 6 others remained hospitalized.

- March 11, 2006, Fleurus, Belgium: an operator working for the company Sterigenics, a medical equipment sterilization site, entered the irradiation room and remained there for 20 seconds; the room contained an unshielded source made of Co-60. When not in use it must be stored in a way that provides shielding from the radiation energy. In this case, the company used water submersion to provide the necessary shielding, allowing safe entry into the room. Three weeks later, the worker developed symptoms typical of irradiation (vomiting, loss of hair, fatigue). One estimate that he was exposed to a dose of between 440 and 480 roentgen equivalent man (REM) because of a malfunction of the control-command hydraulic system maintaining the radioactive source in the pool. The operator spent more than 1 month in a specialized hospital before going back home. To protect workers, the federal nuclear control agency L'Agence fédérale de Contrôle nucléaire (AFCN) and private auditors from the Association Vincotte Nuclear (AVN; a Belgian private nonprofit organization that researches radiochemistry, materials, nuclear medicine, and so forth) recommended Sterigenics to install a redundant system of security.

- February 2011, New Jersey: a chemist killed her husband with a radioactive poison to avoid going through a divorce, prosecutors have claimed. Tianle Li is suspected of giving her husband Xiaoye Wang deadly doses of thallium. The 39-year-old computer engineer, who lived with his wife and 2-year-old son in Middlesex County, New Jersey, thought he had flu when he checked into the University of Princeton Hospital. Doctors were unable to determine what was wrong with Mr Wang, until a nurse remembered a case more than a decade ago when she read about a student in China who died of thallium poisoning. Tests confirmed Wang was riddled with the poison, but by the time the antidote, Prussian blue, arrived, he could not be saved. His 40-year-old widow showed no emotion when she appeared in court to face first-degree murder charges. Tianle is suspected of stealing the poison from the laboratory where she worked at Bristol-Myers Squibb in Lawrenceville, New Jersey.

- November 2009, Kaiga Nuclear Plant, India: Kaiga Generating Station Unit 1, a CANDU (Canada deuterium uranium) reactor design, was shut down for routine maintenance on October 20, 2009. At some point, a water cooler located just outside the reactor building was intentionally contaminated with tritiated water. The lid on the cooler was kept locked. Authorities were able to determine that the contamination was introduced via a drainage/overflow line using a few small vials normally used for sampling the heavy water contained in the primary cooling loop of the reactor. It is thought that the individual who deliberately introduced the contamination obtained the vials and the tritiated water after the samples had been analyzed and were thought to have been disposed of. Fifty-five workers reported to the local hospital on November 25 for medical analysis following routine urine bioassays that identified increased tritium levels. The personnel were told to increase their fluid intake and given diuretics to increase the turnover rate of water in their bodies. Two personnel remained at the hospital for additional testing because of the significantly higher tritium levels.

- March 11 to 20, 2011, Fukushima Prefecture, Japan: partial meltdowns in multiple reactors. After the 2011 Tohoku earthquake and tsunami of March 11, the emergency power supply of the Fukushima-Daiichi nuclear power plant failed. This failure was followed by deliberate releases of radioactive gas from reactors 1 and 2 to relieve pressure. On March 12, triggered by decreasing water levels, a hydrogen explosion occurred at reactor 1, resulting in the collapse of the concrete outer structure. Although the reactor containment was confirmed to be intact, the hourly radiation from the plant increased in level. Residents of the Fukushima area were advised to stay inside, close doors and windows, turn off air conditioning, and to cover their mouths with masks, towels, or handkerchiefs, as well as not to drink tap water. By the evening of March 12, the exclusion zone had been extended to 12 miles around the plant and 70,000 to 80,000 people had been evacuated from homes in northern Japan. A second, nearly identical hydrogen explosion occurred in the reactor building for Unit 3 on March 14, with similar effects.

Data from Database of Radiological Incidents and Related Events, compiled by Robert Johnston, Available at http://www.johnstonsarchive.net/nuclear/radevents/index.html.

Radiation

Radiation is simply energy.[1-3] The radiation discussed here is known as ionizing radiation, which is radiation with the energy necessary to remove electrons from their orbits. Radioactive material is the substance that gives off that energy in different forms. It can be compared with fire. The fire in a fireplace gives off heat, a form of energy. The logs and ash in the fire are the material that gives off that energy. When the fire pops and ash is dispersed outside the fireplace, this represents contamination (material outside where it is supposed to be). This material still gives off heat and can be spread throughout the house.

Radiation affects rapidly reproducing cells more than slowly reproducing cells. How this comes into play with treatment and effects is discussed later.

Radiation comes in several forms. This article discusses the most common types and some of their characteristics: alpha, beta, and gamma radiation.

Alpha particles consist of 2 protons and 2 neutrons. On the atomic level, this is a significant-sized particle with a large +2 charge. Because of its size and +2 charge, these particles travel only a short distance before expending all of their energy (usually 3–5 cm). These particles are easily shielded by very thin material, such as paper or the dead layer of human skin cells. This property makes alpha particles harmless outside the body. If people are more than a few inches away from the material emitting alpha radiation, there are no issues. However, if the material is ingested or inhaled and the radioactive material is in contact with the cell linings of the lungs or gastrointestinal tract, the same is not the case. Alpha particles are emitted from naturally occurring materials (eg, uranium, thorium, and radium) and man-made elements (eg, plutonium and americium). These alpha emitters are primarily used (in very small amounts) in items such as smoke detectors.

Beta particles are small −1 charged particles the size of electrons. Smaller and faster, these particles travel 1.2 to 3 m (4 – 10 feet), depending on their energy level. The beta particles can be shielding by plastic the thickness of a credit card or a thin sheet of aluminum. In sufficient quantities with high energy levels and prolonged exposure, they may cause cataracts and skin burns. Beta particles are emitted from naturally occurring material such as stromtium-90. Beta emitters are used in medical applications, such as treating eye disease.

Gamma or x-ray radiation consists of photon energy. It has no mass or charge. It may travel 10s of meters and needs a substance such as concrete for shielding. For that reason, gamma rays such as those emitted by cobalt-60 are often used to treat cancer or sterilize medical equipment. Similarly, x-rays are used to provide images of body parts such as teeth and bone, and in the industrial setting to discover defects in welding operations.

Radiation and its Effects

People are exposed to radiation every day of their lives. Cosmic radiation comes from outer space. Radiation is commonly introduced to humans from radon gas, from natural elements within the Earth's crust, and the plants and animal that people eat, and everyone has a radioisotope that occurs naturally in the body. These types are forms of natural background radiation. There are also man-made radiation sources. Examples of such are discharges from power plants, medical and dental procedures, television sets, and cigarettes.

According to the *National Council on Radiation Protection and Measurement (NCRP) Report 160*, in the United States, people receive about 0.62 roentgen equivalent man (REM) or 620 mrem/y from all sources[4] (natural background and man made). It is common for people to receive far more than 620 mrem in a given year if they have any medical procedures performed. Compare this with the annual allowed dose for a radiation worker in any field, which is 5000 mrem/y.

Exposure to a significant dose of radiation in a short period of time is an acute exposure and may cause detrimental effects. The more clinicians understand about the effects, the better they can evaluate the risk and benefits associated with exposure.

Where do these data come from? Scientists began to collect and analyze information about the biological effects of ionizing radiation shortly after its discovery. Although there is little concrete evidence of the effects from low doses of radiation, scientists have predicted effects based on studies of individuals and groups that have received large doses of radiation. These groups include earlier radiation workers, 80,000 survivors of the atomic bombs dropped in Hiroshima and Nagasaki, patients from radiation accidents such as in Chernobyl, patients with cancer, and several small-scale irradiator accidents.

So, what does the radiation do to human cells? Radiation causes damage to living material by ionizing the atoms in that material: changing the atomic structure of the material. When atoms are ionized, the chemical properties are altered, which changes the resulting chemical behavior. Natural background radiation was mentioned earlier. Does it not also alter the atoms, cells, and molecules? Yes, but at a rate at which bodies can repair the damage as needed.

Radiation affects rapidly reproducing cells more than cells that reproduce slowly. Examples of rapidly dividing cells include blood-forming cells (bone marrow); stem cells, which are more primitive and also more sensitive; and the cells lining the intestinal tract. Again, the primitive crypt cells are more sensitive than the more mature epithelial cells. Also, the cells in embryos or fetuses are uniquely vulnerable to ionizing radiation.

Cells that divide more slowly are thus more resistant to the effects of ionizing radiation, such as muscle cells, nerve cells, and brain cells.

The biological effects of ionizing radiation depend on how fast a radiation dose is delivered and how much is received. An acute radiation dose is a large amount of radiation received in a short period, and a chronic radiation dose is small amount of radiation received over a long period of time. Chronic radiation doses are more common because this is the primary dose received by radiation utility workers, medical personnel, and those in research.

Recognizing the Radioactive Hazard

When responding to a call with injuries, how can radioactive materials be identified? The same way that any other hazards are identified. Radioactive material is listed as class 7 hazardous waste by the Department of Transportation. The level of material dictates the labeling. Most, if not all, first response organizations carry the *Emergency Response Guidebook* (ERG), published by the Pipeline and Hazardous Materials Safety Administration, a division of the Department of Transportation, which provides first responders with a go-to manual to help deal with hazmat transportation accidents during the critical first 30 minutes (https://www.phmsa.dot.gov/hazmat/erg/emergency-response-guidebook-erg).

Patient Handling

Most clinicians have handled a contaminated patient.[5] Contamination is a broad term. This article discusses radiative material contamination, but patients covered with blood are also contaminated. Patients who have been involved in a chemical release are also considered contaminated. Clinicians protect themselves from radioactive contamination the same way they protect themselves from any other contaminant.

Universal precautions are needed while treating these patients. The Occupation Safety and Health Administration defines universal precautions as an approach to infection control to treat all human blood and certain human body fluids as if they were known to be infectious for human immunodeficiency virus, hepatitis B virus, and other blood-borne pathogens (Blood borne Pathogens Standard 29 CFR 1910.1030(b) definition). More information can be found at their health care e-tools Web site, https://www.osha.gov/SLTC/etools/hospital/hazards/univprec/univ.html.

Do not delay treatment of a life-threatening injury or condition. The ERG mentioned previously states that critical or emergency patient care takes priority over radiological assessment or decontamination. If condition or injury permits, then decontaminate as much a possible but do not delay treatment of life-threatening injuries.

In general, there are 3 classes of patients that can be encountered when radioactive material is involved. Patients who have been exposed to radiation from an external source (external irradiation), patients with external radioactive contamination, and patients with internal radioactive contamination (incorporation). Each case and the precautions to take are discussed next.

External Source (External Irradiation)

There are many ways that patients can be exposed to radiation from an external source. Chest radiograph (x-rays) is an example of external exposure. Another example with different results is cancer treatment. A target area is exposed to a significant amount of radiation with the intent to kill cancer cells. These exposures are planned. An example of an unplanned exposure is an irradiator facility that has experienced a safety malfunction allowing a source to be exposed when workers are in the area. Such patients are not contaminated. They have been near a radioactive source and exposed to a large amount of radiation energy. Once they are removed from the area of the radiation source, there is not a radiological hazard to the responder. Depending on the amount of radiation dose received, which can be shown on a self-reading dosimeter, which radiation workers are required to wear, these patients may need immediate transport to a medical facility for treatment. A sudden onset of nausea and vomiting is an indication of an acute high level of radiation exposure.

External Radioactive Contamination

This topic is discussed in *Medical Management of Radiological Casualties*, by the Armed Forces Radiobiology Research Institute[5] (AFRRI Special Publication 10-1, fourth edition, 2013).

External radioactive contamination refers to radioactive material deposited on a patient's skin and clothing. Examples include radiation workers injuring themselves while working in a contaminated area, such as in a nuclear power plant or a laboratory. Another example is a traffic accident involving a vehicle transporting low-level radioactive material. This type of contamination is the easiest to remove. These patients require universal precautions to protect the responders. The contamination levels are highly unlikely to be at a level at which they pose a radiation exposure hazard to caregivers. However, the situation must be handled to minimize the cross-contamination of the ambulance or other transport, and this is easily done with a few steps. If possible, remove the patient's outer layer of clothing. The items removed from the patient need to be in a container, such as a plastic bag, that is identified as radioactive material. This container could also be labeled as a biohazard as needed. This step removes a significant portion of the contamination. Place 1 or 2 sheets over the stretcher, place the patient on the sheets, then wrap the sheets around the patient to contain contaminants. Only leave exposed the face and any part of the body that may need medical attention. Change gloves often. Not only does this protect the provider, it reduces the amount of time required to clear the transport vehicle to return to service. If the equipment is available, survey the mouth and nose area for external contamination, which is done with handheld radiation detection equipment. Take a swab of the nasal passage, have the individuals blow their noses and survey the results, and perform a direct frisk of the area of the mouth and nose. Positive results (ie, indication of the presence of radioactive material) inside the mucosal region indicate an increased likelihood of internal contamination.

Internal Radioactive Contamination: Incorporation

Patients with internal radioactive contamination pose little threat to responders. Internal contamination refers to radioactive material that has entered the body through a portal of entry. The material can in ingested, inhaled, absorbed, or injected, such as in an impaled injury. These patients may need medical intervention to enhance the process of ridding the body of the radioactive material. For this, clinicians need to know the isotopes that have entered the body (this is discussed further in relation to patient treatment).

It was mentioned earlier that the radiation dose limit for workers is 5 REM or 5000 mrem/y. This amount is the limit for the total effective dose equivalent, which is defined by the Nuclear Regulatory Commission as the sum of the effective dose equivalent (external exposure) and the committed effective dose equivalent (internal exposure). Per the National Health Physics Society, radiogenic health effects such as the damage to cells have not been observed at less than 10 REM or 10,000 mrem of dose received.

Facility Preparation

An emergency radiation/treatment area and an ambulatory decontamination area should be designated along with protocols in place to respond to patients exposed to radiation.[6] The area should be of sufficient size and layout. It should have only 1 pathway to enter and exit. It should be situated so as to have a minimal impact on the operations of the emergency department. Ideally, that area should have 2 boundaries. A so-called hot zone for the treatment area, a warm zone to process personnel and equipment into and out of the treatment area, and a cold zone. Items and personnel that exit the warm zone to the cold zone have been surveyed and are considered as released. No further actions are required.

Hot Zone or Treatment Area

This area is equipped to treat ill or injured patients who also have radioactive contamination. This area is specifically designed or constructed as a decontamination/treatment area or is an area that is temporarily retrofitted to prevent the spread of contamination, such an existing treatment or trauma room.

The treatment area is stocked with personal protective equipment (PPE) to protect the health care workers and to prevent the spread of contaminants. This equipment includes, but is not limited to, eye protection glasses with side shields or eye and face shield combinations, and N-95 airborne mask. This equipment provides some protection against the potential for airborne radioactive material. Disposable gowns (eg, Tyvek) and latex gloves are also needed (note: wearing 2–3 pairs allow clinicians to change gloves as needed). If gloves are changed while in the ambulance, place the potentially contaminated gloves in a bag for monitoring and disposal. Nonporous shoe covers and head covering are also of high utility.

Ambulatory Decontamination Area

The ambulatory decontamination area is for patients that are either not injured or minimally injured but have external radioactive contamination. Essentially a shower is all that is needed where patients can perform self-decontamination with guidance from the staff to shower as they normally would, being careful to not allow shower water to enter the mouth or nose, and outer clothing to be discarded.

Other considerations concerning the treatment/decontamination area are much like those for any treatment area.

- Is there an adequate water supply?
- Can the water be heated as needed?
- Is the drainage contained (holding tanks of sufficient volume) to not contaminate the outside areas?
- Is there adequate lighting?
- Does the ventilation system have the necessary filtering in place?
- Is there a public-address system to clearly and effectively communicate?

These requirements are some, but not all, of the needs of the treatment area, but are a good start.

Patient Treatment

Internally contaminated patients

There are 4 strategies for removal of internal radioisotopes. The treatment depends on the chemical nature of the isotope. Some patients have rapid incorporation or toxicity properties that call for treatment because of suspicion of internal contamination.[5]

These 4 strategies are isotopic dilution, decreasing the absorption from the gastrointestinal tract, blocking incorporation, and mobilizing agents (**Box 2**). These treatment processes are intended to decrease the amount of time that a radioisotope is in the body. The isotope has a radiological half-life, which is the amount of time for half of

---

Box 2
Four strategies for removal of internal radioisotopes

- Isotopic dilution. An example of this is tritium in the form of tritiated water. By administering large amounts of the stable forms of the isotope, the body flushes by normal means. The fluids can be given orally or intravenously. The body does not differentiate between H_2O water and H_3O tritiated water. Diuretics can also be used if needed.

- Decrease the absorption from the gastrointestinal tract by decreasing the solubility so the material passes through with the stool. Removing the material from the stomach by gastric lavage also accomplishes decreased absorption. Other methods include barium sulfate (oral contrast dye), which creates insoluble sulfates of strontium and radium. Prussian blue (Radiogardase) binds with cesium and thallium, aluminum, and magnesium salts (Maalox or Mylanta) reduce the absorption of radium and strontium.

- Block incorporation. When the target organ is saturated with a stable form of the isotope it cannot take up any more. The best example of this is with iodine and the thyroid. Of the 37 different isotopes of iodine,[7] only iodine-127 is stable, and this is the substance in the potassium iodine tablets (radiation pills) that can be issued after a nuclear plant accident. Remember that, once the target organ is flooded with the stable isotope, it needs to be kept flooded until the threat is minimized.

- Mobilizing agents, such as those used in chelation therapy, enhance the elimination of materials from the body. Radioactive isotopes such as manganese, plutonium, and americium are excreted slowly, if at all, by the kidneys. Chelating agents such as diethylenetriamine pentaacetate and ethylenediaminetetraacetic acid form compounds with these metal that make them easier to excrete.

Data from DOE Modular Emergency Response Radiological Transportation Training and FEMA Hospital Emergency Department Management of Radiation Accidents.

the substance to decay to another form. There is nothing that can change this. However, there is also a biological half-life, which is the amount of time it takes the body to process and eliminate half of the substance. The rule to follow is that, after 7 half-lives, less than 1% of the original substance remains. After 10 half-lives, less than 0.1% of the substance remains.[8,9]

All of these treatment methods have 1 thing in common: they are medical treatments and, as such, are to be performed in a controlled environment by knowledgeable licensed health care providers. As with any treatment, monitoring of results is crucial.

Externally contaminated patients

This article does not discuss how to treat an illness or injury but discusses how to deal with patients who have external contamination. As mentioned earlier, people cannot detect radioactive material with their senses. Clinicians treat according to the report given to them by either the emergency providers delivering the patients or by the patients themselves. The process of decontaminating the patients and preventing the spread or cross-contamination is key. This process can be repetitive because not all the contaminants may be removed with the first attempt. Some guidelines follow.

Begin with the careful removal of clothing. Depending on the situation, removal of clothing removes a portion of the contamination. In Wisconsin in February, this would be a significant portion of the contamination. In South Beach in Miami, Florida, in July, it may not be so much. An individual trained to do so, such as the staff radiation safety officer, surveys the patient to identify the area and levels of contamination. This survey is performed using a count-rate instrument for a direct frisk of the patient performed by the trained individual; routine medical personnel do not perform this task. Also, samples such as swabs, smears, and possibly used dressings need to be labeled with patient data, location of the sample, the time taken, and when in the decontamination process the sample was taken. These samples are checked for radioactivity and then sent to a laboratory for isotope identification.

The priorities of decontamination depend on the situation. A guideline to follow is to decontaminate areas of entry (wounds, mouth, nose, eyes, and ears) first to reduce the possibility of internalization. Areas of higher contamination should be addressed before areas of lower contamination.

Decontaminate a wound in the same way as any wound would be cleaned. Attention must be paid to not cross contaminate or spread contamination. Channel fluids to a container if possible; do not spill it on the floor. Gentle irrigation with sufficient amounts of water or saline should remove most of the contamination. A hydrogen peroxide or Betadine surgical scrub may be needed.

When to stop decontamination efforts depends on the results of the decontamination efforts. A guide to follow is to stop decontamination efforts if, after many attempts, the contamination level ceases to decrease, the decontamination efforts are causing damage to the patients, and/or the area is determined to be free of contaminants.

Clinicians' Perspective in Radiation Response

Initial thoughts on radiation casualties should flow along 2 pathways, which concern the incident as well as the patient. Incident medical response emphasis is targeted toward removal from radiation sources, reduction in contamination spread, patient decontamination, field dosimetry, and identification of casualties who initially appear well but who require delayed lifesaving interventions. Patient medical approach is very basic and includes lifesaving measures, decontamination, and nonemergent medical interventions performed with consultation by health physics experts. The mobile app REMM (Radiation Event Medical Management) can also help aid providers.

Event-oriented Medical Approach

At the scene, the questions concern the number of people exposed or contaminated. If there is an isolated casualty in an environment such as an industrial irradiator, where 1 person stepped beyond a safe line, the variables reduce because the event is an isolated patient who is exposed, not contaminated. In the event that there is a dispersal device of sorts, with multiple patients involved, layers of complexity are added because the risk for delayed-onset illness of exposed patients arises. It is very common in large events for standard emergency medical service triage to dismiss well-appearing and well-feeling persons at the scene of an event. In a large-scale radiation emergency, it is key to contain people who were within the venue in which the event occurred. The justification for such containment is that the walking well may have been exposed to a dosing of energy radiation significant enough to produce hematopoietic syndrome without other initial symptoms. This dosing is greater than 1 Gy but is of almost definitive risk at a dose greater than 2 Gy.[10,11] Appropriate on-scene emergency medical service response before local radiation health expert arrival should be to quarantine these individuals, monitor the percentage of the patient's vomit, measure the time from the exposure until each individual vomited, and a by-name pinpoint on a map of the venue where the individuals were located. This work serves the purposes of assisting in locating the center point of the exposure as well as assisting with field dose estimations. Reachback to Radiation Emergency Assistance Center/Training Site (REAC/TS) at 865-576-1005 (24 hours a day) with percentage emesis and time to emesis data provides clinicians and field responders with rapid dosimetry estimations (**Box 3**).

Once a registry of exposed patients, field dosimetry, and decontamination are concluded, asymptomatic individuals with dose estimations less than 0.5 Gy may be followed up through public health and primary care channels with serial complete blood counts (CBCs) with differential to assess for onset of hematopoietic syndrome. Those with radiation doses greater than 0.5 Gy should have a baseline CBC with differential drawn with biweekly follow-ups coordinated to ensure that radiation-induced bone marrow suppression has not initiated pancytopenia to the extent that would require transfusions.

Patient-oriented Medical Approach

There are no documented injuries to care providers of radiation-contaminated casualties, which should provide comfort to clinicians but not to the degree that would

---

Box 3
Key points for on-scene medical response

- Triage all persons and treat/evacuate those requiring lifesaving measures
- Quarantine all nonemergent patients within vicinity of the event who have been exposed or contaminated
- Collect and map individual data on locations within the venue of the event
- Identify all patients who vomit within specific period of time between the event and the episode of emesis
- Calculate the percentage of those in the venue who have shown symptoms of emesis
- Decontaminate nonemergent patients and ensure patients are followed for potential cytopenias

prompt appropriate respiratory and mucosal membrane protections along with a dosimetry device if one can be obtained. In addition, pregnant clinicians should use greater precautions in avoiding radiation exposures. Given that treating radiation-contaminated patients while wearing PPE is generally safe, lifesaving treatments both in and out of hospital are to be performed before decontamination. This guideline is in distinction to chemical and biological casualties, who must be decontaminated first. However, this does not mean that nonemergent casualties or walking-well patients do not require appropriate decontamination and monitoring, to include alpha and beta particle assessments of wounds and nasal swabs for verification. Once emergency procedures and all anticipated surgeries are conducted, emphasis can be then be directed toward wound decontamination, isotope identification, and treatment measures for remaining injuries performed in conjunction with consultation with health physics experts. Of note, because of likely pancytopenia starting with immune cellular lines, it is important to conduct surgeries that may be required due to trauma or illness which may or may not be related to the radiation incident within the first 48 hours of initial injury.[10] Hospitals are likely to be flooded with people showing symptoms of anxiety and emesis secondary to anxiety caused by the reports of a radiation incident. A streamlined process of assessing these potential patients would prevent hospitals from becoming overwhelmed to the extent that they cannot manage the sick and wounded that require care. In addition, many radioactive metals are also water reactive. It serves clinicians well to conduct dry debridement of visible substances before flushing wounds.

Clinicians approaching these situations with the appropriate level of tactical patience and assertiveness need to stick to the basic principles of medicine. Appropriate PPE to protect mucosa from internal contamination of radioactive substances must be remembered. Lifesaving measures precede decontamination. Well-appearing and healthy-feeling patients may still require delayed medical intervention. When in doubt, call health physics for reachback, and REAC/TS is available 24 hours a day, 7 days a week, to assist with navigating these problems.

Clinicians cannot know all the answers. They can know where to reach out to for help. The following is a brief list of resources. Check with local and state jurisdictions for availability.

REAC/TS
https://orise.orau.gov/
US Government Department of Health and Human Services REMM
https://www.remm.nlm.gov/
Centers for Disease Control and Prevention (CDC), emergency preparedness and response
https://emergency.cdc.gov/
Radiation Injury Treatment Network (RITN)
https://ritn.net/
The National Health Physics Society.
http://www.hps.org

REFERENCES

1. DOE Modular Emergency Response Radiological Transportation Training.
2. FEMA Hospital Emergency Department Management of Radiation Accidents.
3. DOE RCT Handbook, DOE-HDBK-1122-99.
4. National Council on Radiation Protection and Measurement (NCRP) Report 160.
5. Medical Management of Radiological Casualties, Armed Forces Radiobiology Research Institute. AFRRI Special Publication 10-1, 4th addition, 2013.

6. American College of Radiology. Disaster preparedness for radiology professionals 2006. US Government: Government version 3.0.

7. Available at: https://www.sciencedirect.com/topics/immunology-and-microbiology/isotopes-of-iodine. Accessed May, 2019.

8. Los Alamos Radiation Monitoring Handbook, James T Voss, NRRPT, CHP, Fellow of the Health Physics Society 2011 update.

9. Seventeenth edition nuclides and isotopes: chart of the nuclides. Knolls Atomic Power Lab; 2010.

10. McFee RB, Leikin JB. Toxico-terrorism : emergency response and clinical approach to chemical, biological, and radiological agents. New York: McGraw-Hill, Health Professions Division; 2008.

11. Sugarma SL, Goans RE, Garrett AS, et al. The medical aspects of radiation incidents. Oak Ridge (TN): Oak Ridge Associated Universities; 2011.

Pathogens and Toxins of High Consequence

Category A and B Agents and Synthetic Biology: A Practical Guide to Understanding

Nathaniel J. Taylor, MPAS, PA-C[a],*,
Stephan C. Kesterson, MPAS, PA-C[b]

KEYWORDS

- CDC level A • CDC level B • Bioterrorism • Anthrax • Smallpox • Botulism
- Tularemia • Viral hemorrhagic fevers

KEY POINTS

- Biological agents are a legitimate threat for state-level warfare and rogue actor terror.
- There are key clinical features of most of these conditions that indicate their likelihood with specific definitive diagnostics and treatments available for each.
- Although it is difficult to maintain a suspicion for these biological agents, multiple patients presenting at the same time with atypical symptoms should prompt early engagement of public health authorities.
- Modern advancements in engineering technology are revolutionizing the world creating the potential for both amazing and catastrophic outcomes in the biological world.

INTRODUCTION

The use of biological agents to incapacitate or kill a perceived enemy dates back before when the perception of the microbiological world, as we know it, developed. Suggested early uses of biological warfare exist with the potential use of Clostridium-coated arrows by Scythian archers in the Trojan war (<1000 BCE) as well as several instances of well-water pollution and city catapult assaults with microbe-infested bodies at the hands of the tyrants and conquerors of history. In more modern history such as the 1700s, the British Crown ordered blankets used by patients infected with smallpox to be distributed among American natives. Just

[a] 91st Weapons of Mass Destruction Team, 5636 E. McDowell Road, M203, Phoenix, AZ 85008, USA; [b] Expeditionary Medical Decontamination Team, 2501 Capehart Road, Omaha, NE 68133, USA
* Corresponding author.
E-mail address: nathaniel.j.taylor16.mil@mail.mil

Physician Assist Clin 4 (2019) 727–738
https://doi.org/10.1016/j.cpha.2019.06.002
2405-7991/19/Published by Elsevier Inc.

within roughly the last hundred years, one may observe instances such as the Germans infecting allied nation livestock with Anthrax and Glanders (a potentially fatal systemic illness for horses) and the Japanese government dispersing plague and other pathogens across China.[1,2]

Biological methodology as a platform of attack stands unique amongst its peers of radiological, chemical, and conventional methodologies due to multiple factors. First and foremost, the inability to contain the spread of a biological pathogen makes the utilization of these agents something that requires more planning and consideration. This, combined with latent onset of symptoms or "latency," compounds these considerations. As an example, the incubation period for avian influenza is around 5 days with some cases ranging up to 17 days. People transmit influenza from 1 day before symptoms all the way through their full onset of sickness, which is roughly 5 days after onset of symptoms. As an example, if a terror entity weaponized avian influenza to spread from person to person with the intent of harming an enemy while protecting their own people, they would have to account for all of the contacts of patient zero as well as their down-the-line contacts ad infinitum. With modern speed of travel this type of epidemiologic mapping is not only exceptionally difficult but also depends on virulence factors of the pathogen that vary and in the case of a quiet hastily reworked avian influenza would likely be unavailable. Although these factors are legitimate reasons to avoid biological weapons as a platform of attack, they do not negate the possibility of a highly sophisticated state-level weapons attack, a fatalist regime biological weapon, or a rogue terror organization willing to sacrifice their own to achieve a terror objective. These characteristics are unique to biological pathogens opposed to toxins due to the fact that toxins in many ways behave like chemicals in that they are not alive and do not replicate.

The diversity of options for the development of potential weaponized biological agents is as complex as the microbiological world. The Center for Disease Control (CDC) established a triage system of sorts that risk stratifies potential biological warfare agents based on the simplicity of dissemination, difficulty of identification, associated mortality rates, and ability to create panic in a population. They categorize these in categories A, B, and C with "CDC Category A" agents being those of most concern. In total, the 3 categories have 20 agent categories that would require volumes of work to address in any exhaustive manner. Here, the emphasis will prioritize Category A and B agents and then address treatment concepts that are applicable across the spectrum of treatment of victims of weaponized biological agents.

Category A Agents

Smallpox virus

Smallpox (variola) is a viral pathogen of special note for multiple reasons. It is a naturally occurring virus that is unique to humans. There are dozens of recognized poxviruses that are unique to a specific species or a group of similar species. Some are unique to cows, chickens, mollusks, etc. In the process of epidemiologic research on smallpox outbreaks, it was noted that people milking cows for work had survived specific regional smallpox outbreaks. On further study it was noted that these people had come into contact with cowpox and thus derived immunity to smallpox. This brought about the change from the former process of "variolation," the process of snorting smallpox scabs from victims in order to derive immunity, to "vaccination" with vaccinia, which created a pox lesion at the injection site in immunocompetent hosts. Of historical note, this was both the original vaccine and the basis for the nomenclature vaccination.[1] With an effective vaccine and control measures put into place, naturally occurring smallpox was eradicated as of 1978. This fact alone makes much of the modern treatment approaches to smallpox infections theoretic in nature. After a few laboratory incidents, all smallpox viruses in laboratory settings were theoretically destroyed, with the only laboratories still maintaining the virus being the CDC in Atlanta and the Vector Institute in Russia. As such, any suspected case of smallpox must be reported through both public health channels and the Federal Bureau of Investigation as it would be considered a nefarious cause case.

Patients with smallpox appear sick with fevers and a series of pustules throughout the body all in the same stage of development unlike chickenpox. In addition, these pustules extend into the palms of the hands and soles of the feet, which put it into a narrower differential along with things such as syphilis, hand-foot-and-mouth disease, Rocky Mountain spotted fever, and few others. These lesions in conjunction with other lesions disseminated throughout the body, mental status changes, and others in the waiting room with similar symptoms would largely suggest the diagnosis.[1,2] Because of the extreme virulence of smallpox, initial personal protection must include respiratory, skin, and mucosal protections for clinicians as well as negative pressure isolation for individuals exhibiting symptoms. Preventing spread of infection will be of greater utility than speedily treating a solitary individual or small group. Anyone who had been in open air contact or shared ventilation with the individual will need to be isolated and quarantined away from those who have not for public health interface until all their scabs fall off. Those with fevers should be again separated from that group and the clinical facility will need to be placed on divert. Tissue specimen collection techniques can be obtained in the Department of Defense Smallpox Response Plan in an open source format through the Department of Homeland Security Website: https://www.hsdl.org/?abstract&did=441826. In addition to isolation and pursuit of accurate diagnosis through laboratory analysis individual treatments consisting of vaccinia immune globulin intramuscularly and/or intravenously may be of some benefit with a preference for the intravenous option. Postexposure vaccination with standard smallpox vaccine may improve outcomes as well. Antivirals that have shown the greatest potential for efficacy in mitigating the effects of smallpox are Tecovirimat, Cidofovir, and Brincidofovir. Immune globulin and antivirals for the treatment of smallpox are readily available at strategic locations throughout the country and can be accessed through public health channels.[2] In addition, there is a reservoir of vaccines that are accessible through the Department of Defense as they still maintain an active smallpox vaccination program.

Bacillus anthracis (anthrax)

Anthrax in many regards is the paradigmatic state-level biological weapon of attack. Bacillus anthracis is easily accessible in nature from soil particularly near livestock, and with high-level microbiological work, it can be made into a weapon of exceptional capability to spread quickly and inflict a lot of damage on people while contaminating a great area with hardy spores. Bacillus anthracis in its live state can be exposed to limited common antibiotic treatments to develop resistance patterns to the antibiotics traditionally indicated for its treatment as outlined later. Its spores can be isolated to specific micron sizes to remain in the terminal alveoli in the lungs as opposed to those too small that may be exhaled or those too large that would be caught in the gastrointestinal system or upper airways and it can be affixed to silica to permit longer suspension in the air. These are just a small number of processes of "heating up" this agent to inflict more damage on unsuspecting populations. Domestic attacks with anthrax are a part of the not-too-distant past of the United States. In 2001 anthrax was used by way of letter-mail for the purposes of terror, which resulted in 22 confirmed or suspected cases of anthrax. Of the half of these that were inhalational cases, 5 died. The remaining cases were cutaneous and more than 33,000 people required postexposure prophylaxis, which is 60 days of either doxycycline or ciprofloxacin along with a 3-dose regimen of anthrax vaccine.[2] The response and mitigation of this incident ranged in the billions of dollars all stemming from 5 letters. Now it is understood that the person who opened the letter in the Hart Senate Office Building recognized the powder and set the letter down before alerting authorities. Just from that amount of movement and the spore's permeation of the pores on the letter, the spores were identified both several stores up and several stores down from the floor it was identified on. It is widely accepted with some controversy that the anthrax that was used in these attacks originated from United States biological countermeasures laboratories. Without a doubt, scientifically speaking, the characteristics of the anthrax would be used to identify it as a state-level product, which means there are other potential high-end modifications to the bacteria and spores as a part of a weaponization process. Although nonweaponized anthrax infections do occur, all incidences of anthrax infection within the United States are investigated as if they were of nefarious cause until the FBI and Department of Defense deem it a naturally occurring case.

Two advantages exist for the community at large regarding the use of anthrax as a weapon. Firstly, the process of heating up anthrax to an apex weapon is a state-level process that requires unique expertise and unique financial resources that are not readily available to traditional terror organizations. In addition, once victims with active anthrax symptoms are decontaminated of spores, they present no known risk of transmission from person to person. Human anthrax infection manifests itself in 3 routes: cutaneous, gastrointestinal, and inhalational. It is transmitted from spores coming into contact with these environments that are favorable for germination and growth. Laboratory confirmation of gram-positive bacilli from locations discussed later and colony morphology can be used for presumptive diagnosis in conjunction with clinical signs and symptoms particular to the specific syndromes that are further discussed. Cutaneous anthrax is characteristically a cutaneous ulcer surrounded by fluid-filled vesicles, which over the course of 48 to 72 hours develops into a "black eschar" lesion that falls off in 2 weeks.[1] The fluid-filled vesicle can be used for laboratory specimen collection.

Cutaneous anthrax has about a 20% mortality rate and may be treated with oral Penicillin, although some studies suggest there is no specific benefit to the use of antibiotics for cutaneous anthrax. In addition, cases of coalition force surgeons in Afghanistan performing debridement surgery to remove necrotic tissues and flush the wound have reported positive results. Not enough data exist to indicate that it is better than antibiotic therapy alone or observation.

Gastrointestinal anthrax is rare in humans and is more than likely associated with contaminated meat from naturally occurring spores found on livestock rather than nefarious causes. It presents essentially in the upper digestive tract or lower digestive tract and symptoms mimic inflammatory symptoms of other causes of acute disease in these areas. Diagnosis may prove difficult, as the symptoms of fever, sore throat, dysphagia, cervical lymphadenopathy, nausea, vomiting, and anorexia are very nonspecific. These symptoms in the presence of an anthrax outbreak may be the only indicator to steer a clinician to suspect the diagnosis. Microbiological cultures from the gastrointestinal tract have been ineffective at confirming the diagnosis.

Inhalational anthrax is the most lethal of the infection types, with studies suggesting just 3 spores are all that is required to create clinical disease.[2] The timing of infection after exposure is depends on how long the spores remain dormant before germination within the lungs. Once active disease onsets, patients present with very nonspecific lower respiratory symptoms such as fever, fatigue, and malaise with a nonproductive cough. After a period of several days of symptoms, respiratory demise occurs. Classic chest radiographic findings would include a widened mediastinum, as necrosis and hemorrhage in the perihilar and mediastinal lymph nodes is generated after transport of the bacteria from terminal alveoli in the lungs. Because of rarity, this would likely spark concerns in a trained clinician if there were multiple patients presenting with the same clinical symptoms or a known attack in conjunction with classic radiographic findings.

Both gastrointestinal and inhalational anthrax can manifest similar systemic symptoms and share treatment approaches. Once the disease progresses into septicemia and meningitis, blood cultures may prove useful. Of special note, spinal fluid analysis from anthrax infections that have progressed to meningitis will be hemorrhagic in more than half of the cases and the bacteria can be identified from both culture and microbiology.[1] Mortality in gastrointestinal anthrax infections ranges up to 60% in some studies and treatment should consist of 2 or more antibiotics with a fluoroquinolone or doxycycline and one or more of clindamycin, penicillin, vancomycin, aminoglycosides, imipenem, linezolid, or rifampin.[1] As always, clinicians should coordinate with infectious disease experts and allow susceptibility studies to drive changes to empirical therapy.

Yersinia pestis (plague)

Yersinia pestis is a gram-negative bipolar coccobacillus that transmits disease to humans in nature by way of flea bites. It is naturally occurring in the southwestern United States and intermittently dispersed through all continents except Antarctica and Australia. Classic infections are commonly associated with the lymph nodes nearest to the site of the flea bite becoming inflamed and enlarged approximately 1 to 10 cm in diameter. These nodes and overlaying skin are exquisitely tender and are referred to as "buboes," indicating the classic nomenclature of "bubonic plague." The site of these infections is most commonly inguinal and femoral nodes, given the likely location of flea bites are the lower extremities. However, axillary and cervical chain nodes have also been the heralding buboes in patients who have been flea-bitten in upper extremities. *Y pestis* is a hardy bacterium that has many properties that permit it to evade immune system mitigation and often results in deadly septicemia in most cases with the presence of buboes but not in necessity. The disseminated intravascular coagulopathy (DIC) initiated by the septicemia along with thrombosis of acral vessels results in necrosis and gangrene of the nose, digits, and even extremities.[2] For this reason, plague was often referred to as "black death" during outbreaks of years past. This hematogenous spread of the bacteria may seed in the lungs into a highly contagious variant of *Y pestis* infection known as "pneumonic plague." Although historically the spread of plague was done by dispersing fleas that had fed on infected hosts, the likely form of weaponized plague now exists in aerosolization plague from a liquid base. This would likely make the pneumonic version of plague the initial presentation of the condition rather than buboes. Aside from the presence of buboes, a bloody cough, and acral cyanosis, the symptoms of plague are very generalized and nonspecific, such as fever, generalized lymphadenopathy, DIC, hepatic or splenic tenderness and enlargement, cough, and fatigue. Chest radiographs in pneumonic plague often reveal bilateral infiltrates. Fatality rates in treated bubonic plague have been reported as high as 60%, and there is no substantial evidence that untreated pneumonic plague is survivable. Successful treatment requires early diagnosis, which may prove difficult in patients without the buboes or acral cyanosis. To diagnose bubonic plague, a large syringe with 2 cc of sterile water may be injected into a bubo and the contents of the bubo may be aspirated in order to obtain substance for microscopy/cultures as well as improve symptoms of pain. Septicemic plague may be diagnosed from 3 blood cultures 10 to 30 minutes apart. Pneumonic plague can be diagnosed by simple microscopy/cultures of sputum anywhere in the respiratory tract. A particular benefit for treatment of undiagnosed plague septicemia is that empirical antibiotic therapy is efficacious against standard Y pestis and should either eliminate the disease or prevent mortality until the susceptibility studies yield results.[2] Aminoglycosides, tetracyclines, fluoroquinolones, and chloramphenicol are all effective against natural Y pestis.[1] Consultation with public health and infectious disease experts should be used in order to drive treatment plans.

Botulism toxin
Clostridium botulinum is a naturally occurring pathogen that is 1 of 3 clostridium species that commonly produce "botulism toxin." This is the most lethal biological substance known to mankind. At one point after the Gulf War, Iraq admitted to possessing more than 19,000 L of weaponized botulism toxin, which was enough to annihilate the entire population of the world 3 times over.[2] This condition occurs naturally through spores activating in infant guts from foods such as honey, corn syrup, beans, and varied vegetables or by entering through wounds in the skin or gastrointestinal system. Clostridium botulinum is a gram-positive rod-shaped organism that produces a toxin that inhibits the release of the neurotransmitter acetylcholine across neuromuscular synapses as well as others throughout the body. This results in a descending flaccid paralysis that is associated with preservation of sensation. Inhalational botulism toxidrome is likely the result of a weaponization process. It is often characterized by the presence of diplopia, dysarthria, dysphonia, and dysphagia and a myriad of bulbar palsies.[2] Once the paralysis takes hold, it persists until neural tissue regenerates by way of natural processes. Because of the inhibition of acetylcholinesterase, these patients require significant critical care management. Decompression of an ileus as well as catheterization for urinary retention may be required. Because of the muscles of respiration being paralyzed, these patients require lengthy ventilation until their motor end plate recovers.[1] The toxidrome should be expected with a descending flaccid paralysis especially in the absence of a fever along with the preservation of sensation.[2] Fecal and gastric anaerobic studies can be performed to confirm the diagnosis but these take greater than a week to result. There are however unique electromyogram findings that may indicate the condition such as reduced M-wave amplitudes, excess action potentials, and gradual increase in M-wave amplitudes with repeat stimulation.[1,2] There is an antitoxin for botulism that has been shown to reduce the duration of mechanical ventilation by a significant number of days, which must be accessed through public health channels with little exception. The need for mechanical ventilation is patient dependent and may last several weeks. Given the demand such a condition places on the local medical network, a weaponized dispersal among several victims may quickly overwhelm regional capacity to manage.

Francisella tularensis (Tularemia)
Tularemia is a zoonotic disease that has well over a hundred hosts in nature with no specific identified reservoir. Traditional transmission of Tularemia is typically by way of arthropod bites and the handling of infected small game animals.[1,2] Tularemia has a significant history of weaponization by both the United States and the former USSR. Concerns specifically from the former USSR relate to where specifically their former scientists sought work after the collapse of the Soviet Union. This would lead theorists to suspect the expertise for the weaponization of Tularemia exists in countries who never developed their own research programs. Francisella tularensis is a gram-negative coccobacillus that does not sporulate and has numerous syndromes it may generate from active infection. Of which, the pneumonic version is the most likely manifestation of the illness as a result of a weaponized attack, and

therefore the others will not be addressed in this section. The presentation and chest radiographic findings are very nonspecific but include systemic constitutional symptoms of fever, malaise, weakness, and fatigue. Respiratory examination may be significant for diffuse crackles and pleural rubs in distinction to typical pneumonias. Radiographic findings may indicate apical or miliary infiltrates, and hilar adenopathy is a prominent feature. Otherwise, the diagnosis is something that must be suspected by way of multiple presentations of patients with similar symptomatology. Diagnosis can be achieved with serologic Tularemia tube agglutination testing.[2] Treatment can successfully be achieved with aminoglycosides, tetracyclines, fluoroquinolones, and chloramphenicol.

Viral hemorrhagic fevers

Viral hemorrhagic fevers are arguably the most diverse "agent" contained within the CDC classification system containing viruses from Filoviridae, Arenaviridae, Bunyaviridae, and Flaviviridae families. These enveloped single-strand RNA viruses are notoriously recognized by the nomenclature of the major players in historical outbreaks. Ebola, Marburg, yellow fever, Hanta, West Nile, and Lassa are all just a few of the many names of viruses that rightfully would catch the attention of an astute clinician interfacing with an affected patient population. They make the list of "Level A" concern at the CDC due to the fact that they "are widely distributed in nature and are both stable and highly infectious by airborne means (with some exceptions such as Marburg). They are extremely virulent, have a low infectious dose, and demonstrate a high rate of replication, potentially leading to high morbidity and mortality…".[2] These viruses are contracted classically through insect bites, inhalation, and mucous membrane exposure. They largely involve endothelial infection and thrombocytopenia. The combination of these 2 factors in conjunction with vascular dysregulation generates necrosis and hemorrhage in most organs. Cytokine activation from specific viruses within these families causes significant more vascular permeability and shock.[2,3] The entire class of viral hemorrhagic fevers generates febrile illness along with a myriad of other constitutional symptoms such as nausea, vomiting, and diarrhea. These are often followed by hemorrhage most easily seen in small vessels and mucosa and are accompanied by jaundice and hepatic enlargement. Shock leading to eventual death can occur at rates greater than 90% depending on the agent.[1] Presumptive diagnosis is clinical, and definitive diagnosis can be accomplished by way of Department of Defense/Federal Bureau of Investigation confirmation of weaponized agent or specific virologic studies. Care of these patients is directed toward providing support, preventing secondary infection, pain control, and delirium mitigation. In addition, precautions must be put into place to protect medical and nursing staff. This includes negative pressure isolation with 6 or more air changes per hour, double gloves (leak proof), impermeable gowns, impermeable leg and shoe coverings, face shields, goggles, and N95 cartridge half-faced respirators.[2] Strict attention must be put into place to donning and doffing practices, and decontamination must be in accordance with Environmental Protection Agency standards with specific emphasis on decontamination agent contact time. Immediate showers should be conducted after complete doffing of all clothing and personal protective equipment used in the isolated room with the patient. In a mass casualty situation, open air environments or deeming an entire facility as contaminated may be the only options available to prevent spread of the illness.

Category B Agents

This is the second highest CDC category for biological agents based on acquisition and nefarious dissemination that can lead to moderate morbidity, with a lower rate of mortality compared with Category A agents. These agents are listed in **Box 1**.[3,4]

Brucellosis

Brucella species are considered a zoonotic intracellular aerobic gram-negative cocco-bacillary organism transmitted by an infected host, typically livestock, and may be seen in more domesticated pets such as dogs and some feral animals.[3] The most common form of transmission from animal to human is seen with consumption of undercooked meat and unpasteurized dairy products, although other routes of exposure such as inhalation and direct contact of infected tissue/bodily fluids have been reported, posing occupational and recreational risks.[3] Human-to-human transmission is rare, although vertical transmission can occur in breastfeeding mothers. Its infectivity and aerosol stability led to its weaponization during World War II, becoming the first biological agent weaponized by the United States.[3,5] In aerosolized form, incubatory times can become less latent and effects can be incapacitating compared with its natural state.

There are 4 species of the brucella genus pathogenic to humans—*Brucella abortus*, *Brucella melitensis*, *Brucella suis*, and *Brucella Canis*—each varying in disease manifestation. Incubation periods range from 3 to 4 weeks, although can be as early as 5 days or as latent as months from exposure.[3] Clinical signs and symptoms of brucellosis are seen in **Table 1**.[3,4]

Common physical examination findings include hepatosplenomegaly (10%–70%), arthritis (up to 40%), anorexia, and adenopathy (10%–20%).[3] An index of suspicion should be considered, especially those in endemic areas reporting sacroiliac and testicular pain amongst commonly reported symptoms associated with brucellosis. Additional ancillary support for confirmation includes bone and blood cultures for early

---

Box 1
Category B agents

- Brucellosis (*Brucella* spp.)
- Epsilon toxin of *Clostridium perfringens*
- Food safety threats (*Salmonella* spp., *Escherichia coli* O157:H7, Shigella)
- Glanders (*Burkholderia mallei*)
- Melioidosis (*Burkholderia pseudomallei*)
- Psittacosis (*Chlamydia psittaci*)
- Q fever (*Coxiella burnetii*)
- Ricin toxin (*Ricinus communis*)
- Staphylococcal enterotoxin B
- Typhus fever (*Rickettsia prowazekii*)
- Viral encephalitis (alphaviruses, such as eastern equine encephalitis, and Venezuelan and western equine encephalitis)
- Water safety threats (*Vibrio cholerae, Cryptosporidium parvum*)

Data from Withers MR, Alves DA, U.S. Army Medical Research Institute of Infectious Diseases. USAMRIID's medical management of biological casualties handbook. 8th edition ed. Fort Detrick, Maryland: U.S. Army Medical Research Institute of Infectious Diseases; 2014 and Center for Disease Control and Prevention Emergency Preparedness and Response. Bioterrorism Agents/Diseases. https://emergency.cdc.gov/agent/agentlist-category.asp.

Table 1
Signs and symptoms

- Fever (90%–95%)
- Malaise (80%–95%)
- Sweats (40%–90%)
- Myalgia/Arthralgia (40%–70%)
- GI symptoms (70%)
- Osteoarticular complications (20%–60%)
  - Sacroiliitis (up to 30%)
  - Spondylitis (up to 30%)
  - Lower extremity arthritis (up to 20%)
- Epididymo-orchitis (2%–20%)
- Pulmonary disease (1%–5%)
  - Pulmonary nodules
  - Lung abscess
  - Enlarged hilar lymph nodes
  - Pleural effusion
- CNS invasion (<5%)
- Endocarditis (<2%)

Abbreviations: CNS, central nervous system; GI, gastrointestinal.
Data from Withers MR, Alves DA, U.S. Army Medical Research Institute of Infectious Diseases. USAMRIID's medical management of biological casualties handbook. 8th edition ed. Fort Detrick, Maryland: U.S. Army Medical Research Institute of Infectious Diseases; 2014 and Center for Disease Control and Prevention Emergency Preparedness and Response. Bioterrorism Agents/Diseases. https://emergency.cdc.gov/agent/agentlist-category.asp.

disease, as well as serologic, immunofluorescence, and molecular testing.[3] Other support such as computed tomography/MRI, testicular ultrasound, and electrocardiogram may aid with a suspected diagnosis.[3] Further consultation with an Infectious Disease specialist is warranted for suspected brucellosis in order to adequately treat and identify species from genus. Medical management for acute uncomplicated brucellosis can be found in **Table 2**.[3,5] For complicated brucellosis or relapsing symptoms despite oral antibiotics, seek further treatment options through your Infectious Disease specialists.

Ricin toxin

Ricin is a cytotoxin derived from waste product of castor beans. Its cytotoxic effects inhibit both DNA replication and protein synthesis, leading to cell death.[3] Ricin can be disseminated as a powder, aerosolized, and even injected subcutaneously as suggested regarding the assassination of Georgi Markov in 1978. Although many experts believe that any large-scale use is impractical to achieve a lethal dose, dissemination

Table 2
Medical management for acute uncomplicated brucellosis

Treatment	Duration
• Adults and children >8	4–6 wk
○ Doxycycline, 100 mg, po bid for adults, 2.2 mg/kg po bid (up to 200 mg/d) for children + rifampin 600–900 mg/d po daily for adults, 15–20 mg/kg (up to 600–900 mg/d) for children	
Or	
○ Oral fluoroquinolone (ciprofloxacin/ofloxacin) + rifampin	
Or	
○ Oral TMP-SMX + rifampin	
• Pregnancy and children <8	4–6 wk
○ Oral TMP-SMX + rifampin	

Data from Withers MR, Alves DA, U.S. Army Medical Research Institute of Infectious Diseases. USAMRIID's medical management of biological casualties handbook. 8th edition ed. Fort Detrick, Maryland: U.S. Army Medical Research Institute of Infectious Diseases; 2014 and Teske SS, Huang Y, Tamraker SB, Bartrand TA, Weir MH, Haas CN. Animal and human dose-response models for Brucella species. *Risk Anal* 2011; 31 (10): 1576-96.

on a smaller scale through criminal intent or bioterrorism is a more likely scenario as seen in recent history.[3,6]

Clinical signs and symptoms of ricin poison depend on route of administration and dose. These symptoms have been observed mostly with live tissue models and expected similar in humans based on historical information. Clinical signs and symptoms of ricin poison are seen in **Table 3**.[3,4] Diagnosis can be extremely difficult for pulmonary complaints, as many inhaled biochemical agents elicit respiratory distress, although a large number of similar complaints should prompt early suspicion. Use of ancillary support can provide additional clues to suspected exposure. Given ricin's short half-life and cellular uptake, early detection is critical for confirmation.[3]

Medical management for inhaled ricin exposure is similar to chemical agent exposure with supportive care. Aggressive respiratory support should be administered appropriately for any casualty experiencing respiratory distress. For gastrointestinal intoxication, gastric lavage, volume replacement, and the use of cathartics such as magnesium citrate are current recommendations.[2] Currently there is no vaccination for prophylaxis; however, animal trials continue for preexposure protection.

Staphylococcal enterotoxin B

Staphylococcal enterotoxin B, also known as "SEB," is an exotoxin produced by *Staphylococcus aureus*. There have been no documented cases of intentional release, although this toxin had been weaponized given its potency by weight during the Cold War. SEB was essentially blacklisted in 1970 after President Nixon categorized "toxins" as biological agents during his renounced offensive biological weapon's program in 1969. SEB activity is commonly found with mishandled and contaminated food. Although lethality is low, it can incapacitate causing significant disruption to covert operations, increasing both medical and logistical supportive demands. SEB is considered a "superantigen" that can target and facilitate an inflammatory cascade of cytokines in order to injure host tissue.[3] Symptoms associated with SEB exposure are similar to other biologics, initially presenting with nonspecific influenza as illness symptoms of fever, chills, myalgia/arthralgias, and headache. In severe cases, respiratory distress and retrosternal chest pain may occur.[3] Ingestion

Table 3 Signs and symptoms	

• Inhalation
  ○ Fever
  ○ Sweats
  ○ Cough
  ○ Dyspnea/hyperpnea
  ○ Pulmonary edema
• Injection
  ○ Site necrosis
  ○ Regional lymphadenopathy
  ○ Multiple organ involvement
	• Ingestion
	  ○ Fever
	  ○ Sweats
	  ○ Abdominal pain
	  ○ GI hemorrhage
	  ○ GI, hepatic, splenic, renal necrosis

Abbreviation: GI, gastrointestinal.

Data from Withers MR, Alves DA, U.S. Army Medical Research Institute of Infectious Diseases. USAMRIID's medical management of biological casualties handbook. 8th edition ed. Fort Detrick, Maryland: U.S. Army Medical Research Institute of Infectious Diseases; 2014 and Center for Disease Control and Prevention Emergency Preparedness and Response. Bioterrorism Agents/Diseases. https://emergency.cdc.gov/agent/agentlist-category.asp.

exposure would carry typical gastrointestinal symptoms of nausea, vomiting, abdominal pain, and diarrhea. Typical incubatory times for SEB are 2 to 12 hours postinhalation and 1 to 12 hours postingestion. Symptoms associated with ingestion typically resolve within 24 to 48 hours. Postinhalation resolution may take anywhere from 72 to 96 hours. Use of ancillary support with laboratory work and assays (polymerase chain reaction, enzyme-linked immunosorbent assay using protein AG, electrochemiluminescence) can provide additional clues to suspected acute exposure. Chest radiograph may assist with pulmonary complaints. Treatment of SEB is geared to supportive care. Pulmonary complaints should have appropriate airway management and supplemental oxygen as needed. Volume repletion for gastrointestinal involvement is needed.

Synthetic Biology

Over the past decade, immense changes have taken hold within the biological sciences. More specifically, engineering and computer sciences have set the stage where now real DNA can be assembled based on a computer-based genetic sequence. As more data are collected regarding what specific genetic sequences yield when transcribed, the ability to manipulate, remove, and replace these aspects of a specific DNA chain will manifest. Furthermore, the ability to generate entirely new DNA for a gain of function is permitted with these changes in technology.[7] This process is referred to as "Synthetic Genomics," "Biologic 4-dimensional Printing," or "Synthetic Biology." This process may produce evolutionary changes in what capabilities a human being possess. It generates terrifying possibilities in the realm of bioterrorism. Much of the globe's biosecurity processes are built around a traditional biological world. The DNA for smallpox is maintained at the CDC in Atlanta, GA and the Vector Institute in Russia, yet if someone possessed the genetic sequence information to smallpox in a digital format, they could simply print the virus. The potentials are staggering. If virulence factors such as human-to-human transmission from traditional influenza A were edited into avian influenza, the risk would be pandemic level mayhem. To put that into perspective, modern avian influenza has a mortality rate of 59%. The 1918 influenza pandemic had a mortality rate of a lowly 2.5% and produced more than 50 million deaths.[7] The potential to do such a thing was demonstrated almost 2 decades ago when SUNY researchers synthetically manufactured live polio virus from its DNA sequence in 2002. The level of sophistication required to do this is dramatically decreasing due to technological advancements. What took numerous PhD years to accomplish with $2.7 billion in the sequencing of the genome in 2003 is now so technology dependent that it is farmed out overseas due to lack of domestic profitability costing roughly $100 for the individual. The ordering of genes can be accomplished online for a low rate and modification of DNA sequences is something that can be accomplished in a basic high school science class. The lack of involvement of career biologists brings about the lack of bioethics as this is predominantly a field now led by engineers. On the biosecurity front, there is no way to tell if the next biological outbreak will be traditional or synthetically manufactured, if it was comprised at a national level weapons laboratory or at a local university in the United States or India, or if any of our modeling software, protection, and response measures will be effective against this new threat. The only functional method to confront this reality is through intelligence collection, which is neither perfect nor financially feasible to make comprehensive. The only option for the astute clinician is to remain tuned into disease trends, protect themselves as they were trained, and have a low threshold to involve public health authorities when atypical disease trends emerge.

SUMMARY

Traditional CDC Level A and B agents still are the most likely to be the biological weapon of choice for state warfare and rogue actor terrorism. This is because of the fact that there is the greatest amount of global expertise in these programs, they are stable in a laboratory, and modeling data from natural outbreaks and previous weaponized use provide a degree of predictability once attacks are initiated. Access to aminoglycosides, tetracyclines, chloramphenicol, and fluoroquinolones is key to clinicians in responding to traditional bacterial weapons of attack. Viral pathogens are selected specifically for their ease of transmission from person to person making isolation and proper personal protective equipment use paramount. There are additional agents of concern to the CDC as well as regionally specific threats that must be taken into consideration. It would serve the clinician well to establish a cycle of review to maintain familiarity with these agents, so they may be prepared for the main event when that day comes.

REFERENCES

1. Dembek ZF. Medical aspects of biological warfare. Washington, DC: Borden Institute; 2007.
2. McFee RB, Leikin JB. Toxico-terrorism : emergency response and clinical approach to chemical, biological, and radiological agents. New York: McGraw-Hill, Health Professions Division; 2008.
3. Withers MR, Alves DA, U.S. Army Medical Research Institute of Infectious Diseases. USAMRIID's medical management of biological casualties handbook. 8th edition. Fort Detrick (MD): U.S. Army Medical Research Institute of Infectious Diseases; 2014.
4. Center for Disease Control and Prevention Emergency Preparedness and Response. Bioterrorism Agents/Diseases. Availabe at: https://emergency.cdc.gov/agent/agentlist-category.asp. Accessed March 31, 2019.
5. Teske SS, Huang Y, Tamraker SB, et al. Animal and human dose-response models for Brucella species. Risk Anal 2011;31(10):1576–96.
6. Congressional Research Service. Ricin: Technical Background and Potential Role in Terrorism. Availabe at: https://fas.org/sgp/crs/terror/RS21383.pdf. Accessed March 21, 2019.
7. Garrett L. Biology's Brave New World. Foreign Affairs Magazine 2013.

Terrorist Vehicle Attacks

James E. Patrick, MS, PA-C[a,b,*], Joshua K. Radi, PhD, PA-C[c,d,e,1]

KEYWORDS

- Explosions • VBIED • Ramming • Vehicle • Attack • Terrorism • Medical • Response

KEY POINTS

- Vehicle attacks present a serious terrorist threat to society that requires extreme counter-measures for mitigation and necessitates the appropriate medical response.
- Awareness is at the forefront of detecting and proposing plans and procedures to prevent terrorist activity.
- Knowledge of these types of attacks is gained through prior incidents on the battlefield and developing situational awareness of evolving tactics.

PREFACE

The following is a detailed description by Major Jim Patrick of his firsthand experience involving an attack with the use of a vehicle. This vivid recollection takes place in Iraq, while Major Patrick was deployed with the US Army in support of Operation Iraqi Freedom (OIF). The year 2005 was a period of time in which all of Iraq presented extraordinary challenges for the US military. Whether behind the concrete walls and barriers of a forward operating base (FOB) or patrolling some of the most dangerous roads on earth, soldiers were in constant danger. This day began as another typical scorching hot desert morning and all seemed calm on the FOB 100 km west of Baghdad. The FOB lies within a region known as the Triangle of Death because of the frequency of insurgent attacks on coalition forces. The FOB was located alongside a major thoroughfare that was a highly traveled road used by the US military as well as Iraqi civilian vehicles. Numerous guarded checkpoints were strategically placed along this corridor to thwart insurgent activity.

Disclosure: The views/opinions expressed are those of the authors and do not necessarily represent the views of the Department of the Army and/or the Department of Defense. No other relevant disclosures or conflicts of interest exist.

[a] Medical Detachment, Florida Army National Guard, Starke, FL, USA; [b] Department of Emergency Medicine, Oakes Medical Center, Oakes, ND, USA; [c] 93rd Weapons of Mass Destruction-Civil Support Team, Hawaii Army National Guard, Kapolei, HI, USA; [d] Department of Orthopaedic Surgery, Tripler Army Medical Center, Honolulu, HI, USA; [e] Department of Surgery, University of Hawaii John A. Burns School of Medicine, Honolulu, HI, USA

[1] Present address: 91-802 Launahele Street, Ewa Beach, HI 96706.

* Corresponding author. 10425 Bardin Court, Orlando, FL 32836.

E-mail address: james.e.patrick1.mil@mail.mil

Suddenly, while assessing the missions scheduled for the day at the FOB Tactical Operations Center, a powerful blast echoed through the base and the ground shuddered. One soldier stated, "That was way too close." The explosion occurred at a guarded checkpoint only a short distance away from the FOB. Everyone on the FOB knew that there were American soldiers along with Iraqi soldiers stationed at this checkpoint. Within minutes of the blast, a quick reaction force was deployed to the scene. The horrors of war could not have been more evident on arriving at the checkpoint. It became evident what had occurred. A vehicle-borne improvised explosive device (VBIED) was strategically detonated as it approached the checkpoint.

The US military medical first responders immediately rendered aid to the severely injured soldiers. Car wreckage was scattered about in indistinguishable pieces of twisted metal. Human remains that were hard to differentiate covered the area, and the barely distinguishable body parts were collected. A human forearm and hand were still shackled to the steering wheel, which ultimately had prevented this suicide bomber from not carrying out the mission. The disaster scene investigation entailed trying to determine the number of individuals that had been at the checkpoint and somehow detail the devastation of such a terrorist attack. This VBIED suicide car bombing resulted in the death of 12 Iraqi soldiers and 14 wounded Iraqi soldiers and civilians.

However, this was a horrific event that occurred frequently during OIF. Terrorists and so-called lone-wolf actors have shown the ability to use vehicles as tools for terror not only in Iraq and Afghanistan but internationally and domestically as well. The unfortunate truth is that motor vehicles must be considered as a mode of terror in the wrong hands. This article outlines the different modes in which individuals can use vehicles to attack soft/hard targets, provides guidelines for incident response to medical first responders, and makes recommendations on mitigation efforts that can be used by everyone.

INTRODUCTION

Terrorism is the unlawful use of violence or threat of violence to instill fear and coerce governments or societies. It is often motivated by religious, political, or other ideological beliefs and committed in the pursuit of goals that are usually political.[1] Vehicle terrorism has captivated the world for the past century. In 1920, Buda's wagon, a horse-drawn carriage filled with explosives and scrap metal, was deployed in New York's downtown Manhattan district and left 40 dead and more than 200 injured.[2] Since World War II, society has endured high levels of terrorist activity. In 1972, the Dublin car bombing attack injured more than 100 civilians and the horror was depicted as headlines in all the major newspapers.[3] Western Europe also has a long history of coping with terrorist attacks and subverting concrete plans to undertake such attacks.[4] Ultimately, in the half-century of blast injuries from Northern Ireland to Afghanistan, vehicles have been the weapon of choice during asymmetric warfare.[5]

From 2000 to 2013, Israel had the second highest number of deaths from suicide attacks and was on the list of countries that may experience increases in terrorism because of ongoing conflicts.[6] Israel has encountered numerous vehicle attacks involving both explosives and the ramming of pedestrians, and has become a model for mitigation and emergency medical response.[7] The impact to US military forces during both conflicts in Afghanistan and Iraq continues to set the tone for medical preparation and response to terrorist-based vehicle attacks.

An attack using a vehicle can have many definitions, as this article explains. VBIEDs using automobiles (cars, trucks, vans, transport trucks, semitrailers, buses) are but 1 example, but VBIEDs could potentially be placed in any vehicle, including those on the water or in the air. Similarly, these same vehicles that can be the target of VBIEDs can be used in an alternative manner. For example, planes have been hijacked and used as kamakaze-style missiles, killing everyone onboard the aircraft and having devastating consequences for the area impacted. In addition, automobiles have been hijacked or rented to use as high-speed ramming devices, mowing down any pedestrian or cyclist in their path. Of course, there have been and continue to be many events, as described by Major Patrick, that have targeted military servicemen and women, not just civilians. However, these acts are still inspired by the goal of spreading fear by acts of terror.

An organization dedicated to combating extremism, the Counter Extremism Project (CEP), has documented at least 40 vehicular terrorist attacks on civilians since 2006, which have resulted in 197 people killed and approximately 1066 people injured.[8–10] Terrorist groups that include Al-Qaeda, Hamas, and Islamic State of Iraq and Syria (ISIS) have and continue to use their propaganda machine to promote terrorist attacks using vehicles. In 2010, Al-Qaeda's magazine, Inspire, published a propaganda article requesting new recruits, lone wolves (those with no ties to the terrorist organization), and jihadists to use trucks as weapons. The article was titled "The Ultimate Mowing Machine" and described using a truck as a means to "mow down the enemies of Allah."[11]

As early as 2010, the Federal Bureau of Investigation (FBI) noted that vehicular attacks were becoming an emerging threat, and warned that terrorists had the potential to conduct attacks with minimal prior training or experience.[12] Since this time, there has been a large increase in terrorist attacks using vehicles. Israel in particular, but also Europe and the United States, has seen most of these attacks. Terrorism has changed with the use of vehicles to perform attacks, and the main targets are predominantly Western countries.[13] Propaganda still exists and is a major recruitment tool used by terrorist organizations such as ISIS. In 2016, ISIS publicized another propaganda message via the online magazine Rumiyah. They called for their followers to perform vehicle attacks by targeting "large outdoor conventions and celebrations, pedestrian congested streets, outdoor markets, festivals, parades, and political rallies."[14] ISIS vehicle ramming propaganda from Nashir (a news organization affiliated with ISIS), which aired on a pro-ISIS channel on October 31, 2017.

IMPROVISED EXPLOSIVE DEVICES AND BOMBS

Improvised explosive devices (IEDs), roadside bombs, and suicide car bombs have been responsible for many casualties on the battlefield.[15] IEDs can be made from a wide range of nonmilitary components, chemicals, and compounds that are readily available to civilians in most countries.[16] Because of their improvised nature, the variability in the design, manufacture, and operation of most IEDs defies the traditional paradigms used to assess the effectiveness of conventional munitions.[17]

The IED has therefore been the weapon of choice during asymmetric warfare.[18] Civilian and service personnel casualties cause significant political and social disruption, making the IED a highly profitable asymmetric weapon for insurgent and urban terrorist forces.[19] The result has been an increasing trend worldwide in terrorist bombings. In a viewpoint by Carli and colleagues,[20] the continuing conflicts in the Middle East indicate that many countries around the world will face such situations for many years and medical response not only involves saving lives but also maintains a consistent message that freedom and democracy will never surrender to terrorism designed to instill fear.

These acts can provide lessons and result in improved analysis of terrorist operations and subsequent medical response. The threat area that surrounds an explosion and subsequent blast is determined by the distances any fragments that result from the detonation of the explosive may be expected to travel. During these types of disasters, a basic understanding of explosive blast physics and the associated injury patterns serves as a guide for responding medical personnel to predict medical resources required to perform lifesaving interventions. **Table 1** describes the most common injury patterns seen among explosion survivors.

VEHICLE-BORNE IMPROVISED EXPLOSIVE DEVICES

Terrorists have used vehicles as weapons, or more specifically for weapon transportation, for nearly a century. Since the late twentieth century, the VBIED has been viewed as the most menacing type of weapon in the hands of terrorists.[21] The VBIED currently represents the world's most effective weapon in the hands of terrorists or insurgents, for which even modern armies have no adequate response.[22] This terrorist modality has appeared worldwide and is gradually evolving and modifying so that the effectiveness results in both loss of life and a negative psychological impact on the populace. Converting an easily acquired vehicle into a weapon in order to injure and kill citizens in places where they presume to be safe is the essence and definition of terrorism.[23] When considering a deterrent to this terrorist act, multiple studies show that the VBIED is represented by small cars or light trucks and driven by suicide bombers or a person who has been forced for this purpose. The horror behind suicide VBIEDs is that the enemy is using an expendable human as the targeting hardware.[24]

VEHICLE RAMMING

According to the Transportation Security Administration (TSA), vehicle ramming is defined as "A form of attack in which a perpetrator deliberately aims a motor vehicle at a target with the intent to inflict fatal injuries or significant property damage by striking with concussive force."[25] Supporters of terrorism find vehicle ramming an appealing option because vehicles are easily acquired/accessed, require minimal planning and training, have minimal potential for premature detection, and have the potential to inflict mass fatalities if successful.[26]

Table 1
The most common injury patterns seen among explosion survivors are caused by secondary and tertiary blast injury

Category	Mechanism	Human Injury
Primary	Direct effect of pressurization	Lungs, GI tract
Secondary	Bomb fragments and flying debris	Penetrating trauma
Tertiary	Thrown from blast wave	Blunt trauma and crush injuries
Quaternary	Blast-related injuries, unrelated diseases	Burns, exposure to toxic inhalants, preexisting disease complications

Data from Joseph JW, Sanchez LD. Introduction to Explosions and Blasts. In Ciottone GR. Ciottone's Disaster Medicine, 2e. Philadelphia: Elsevier; 2016, Pages 437-444.

As a nonconventional weapon, the vehicle as a ramming device can be perceived as even more dangerous than explosives. Vehicles are easy to obtain, appear benign, and can wreak devastation to large crowds of people. Terrorist attacks against civilians using a vehicle as a ramming device include potential targets of outdoor assemblies and ceremonies, parades, festivals, political rallies, and crowded inner-city streets.[21] The most recent vehicle ramming attacks have been directed primarily against civilian pedestrians (soft targets) and not necessarily transportation hubs or key figures/leadership (hard targets).[23] The history of vehicles used as ramming devices for terrorist attacks is outlined in **Table 2**.

EMERGING VEHICLE-BASED THREATS

Technological advancements have presented innovative methods of coordinating terrorist activity. Insurgents have quickly adapted to countermeasures, and new, more sophisticated IEDs and vehicle attacks are increasingly being used.[15] Sophisticated modified automobiles now have the ability to be autonomous as a driverless means of transport. Advancements in driverless vehicles have become common among automobile manufacturers and offer the potential for a terrorist attack scenario. In March 2016, FBI researchers presented this risk through remote use of Wi-Fi to access a motor vehicle's electronics and manipulate its function. The threat of driverless VBIEDs and vehicle ramming will be existential when there is a confluence of public use of driverless vehicles in the foreseeable future.[27] Improved understanding of this phenomenon is essential, including how this technology could be applied in a vehicle attack, to then develop countermeasures to preempt such an event.

OPERATIONS, SITE SECURITY, AND INCIDENT RESPONSE

Terrorist vehicle attacks decrease the likelihood of discovery and intervention by authorities before an attack because such an event can be done rapidly and with little preparation.[23] VBIED explosions differ from other explosions because they are common, unpredictable, cause high morbidity and mortality, and are a terrorist method of choice.[28] The question becomes how to recognize, distinguish, and identify potential attack vehicles from nonthreat vehicles. According to Rak and colleagues,[22] the answer is practically nonexistent. Therefore, incidence response preplanning for vehicle-borne terrorist attacks is a key preincident action and must include preestablished coordinated relationships and specified roles between emergency medical service personnel, police, and firefighters.[28] The Department of Defense (DOD) has established the Joint IED Defeat Organization to investigate countermeasures along with various national laboratories, the Department of Energy, contractors, and academia.[15]

In the last decade, the US military and police forces have adopted a new approach for emergency medical care based on an Israeli paradigm that has always been military oriented, with local protocols almost always originating from army milieu.[29] The Israeli first responder community agency entails emergency medical services, police, fire department, military command, and bomb squads. These entities operate in seamless collaboration to decrease casualties and mortality, and provide scene safety. Barriers that withstand a VBIED explosion play a crucial role in protecting important buildings. However, pedestrians and large gatherings of people are often a prime target for terrorism.

Literature shows that militaries acquire a knowledge of a variety of sophisticated mechanisms and deployment strategies from terrorist attacks, thus learning more

Table 2
Historical examples of vehicles used as ramming devices since 2006

Year	Location	Vehicle	Killed	Wounded
2006	University of North Carolina, United States	SUV	0	9
2007	Glasgow Airport, Scotland, United Kingdom	Jeep	0	5
2008	Xinjiang, China	Truck	16	16
	Jerusalem, Israel	Front-end loader	3	40
	Jerusalem, Israel	Bulldozer	0	16
	Jerusalem, Israel	Car	0	19
2009	Jerusalem, Israel	Bulldozer	0	2
2011	Tel Aviv, Israel	Truck	1	17
	Tel Aviv, Israel	Taxi	0	9
2013	Beijing, China	Car	5	0
	London, United Kingdom	Car	1	0
2014	Xinjiang, China	SUV ×2	39	90
	Jerusalem, Israel	Construction tractor	1	5
	Quebec, Canada	Car	1	1
	Jerusalem, Israel	Car	2	7
	Jerusalem, Israel	Car	3	13
	Dijon, France	Car	0	13
	Nantes, France	Car	1	10
2015	Jerusalem, Israel	Car	0	5
	Jerusalem, Israel	Car	1	1
	Graz, Austria	Automobile	3	36
	Lyon, France	Van	1	2
	Jerusalem, Israel	Car	1	2
2016	Valence, France	Car	0	1
	Nice, France	19-ton truck	86	430
	Ohio State University, United States	Car	0	11
	Berlin, Germany	Automobile	12	56
2017	Jerusalem, Israel	Truck	4	0
	London, United Kingdom	Car	5	50
	Stockholm, Sweden	Truck	4	15
	London, United Kingdom	Van	8	48
	London, United Kingdom	Automobile	0	8
	Barcelona, Spain	Van	16	120
	Edmonton, Canada	Car/truck	0	5
	Virginia, United States	Car	1	28
	New York, United States	Home Depot truck	8	12
	West Bank, Israel	Car	0	2
2018	West Bank, Israel	Car	2	2
	London, United Kingdom	Car	0	3
	Danghara, Tajikistan	Car	0	4
	West Bank, Israel	Car	0	3
2019	Tokyo, Japan	Minivan	0	9
	Bottrop and Essen, Germany	Car	0	8
	West Bank, Israel	Car	0	2

Abbreviation: SUV, sports utility vehicle.

during wartime in response to tactical necessities.[24] However, this comes at the expense of casualties during these conflicts. These lessons learned entail a defensive aspect to avoid having an easily acquired vehicle being transformed into a weapon. Transcending the military arena and applying this proficiency to the civilian sector to thwart the strategy and potential consequences of terrorist acts is paramount in the urban environment.

Terrorist vehicle attacks on civilian targets present an upward trend and require consideration for effective countermeasures. Such measures include analysis as to why, when, where, and how these devices were used.[22] Terrorists use VBIED attacks to cause casualties, destabilize societal structure, and bring panic among the civilian population. As the terrorists adapt and innovate to change their tactics, civilian disaster response must remain vigilant for future threats. Vehicles with or without explosives directed against public targets are of utmost concern and attract a great deal of media attention.[23] This media attention offers the benefit of civilian awareness, but it also presents propaganda for the terrorists' cause.

SECONDARY DEVICES AND POSTBLAST CONSIDERATIONS FOR MEDICAL PROVIDERS

A potential pitfall in responding to a terrorist attack is a failure to consider the risk associated with a secondary device after the initial event.[28] Using a secondary device after an explosion of a first device causes confusion and risk to civilians and first responders.

Injuries sustained from an IED can be influenced by many factors, including size, design, and detonation method.[18] The clinical approach taken by medical practitioners to explosive-related injuries depends on the experience of the provider.[30] As a result, the range of injuries and considerations for medical providers requires extensive training and preparation. The clinical approach that medical providers must take into account with explosive-related injuries on arriving at the scene prioritizes casualties with hemorrhage, because exsanguination is of utmost concern.[30] This predominance not only entails trauma life support training for first responders but must also take into consideration an adaptive awareness of secondary devices.

Terrorist attacks in civilian settings tend to have a biphasic distribution of mortality with high immediate rates of death followed by low early and late mortalities, and rarely have civilian providers faced a battlefield approach to triage or sorting.[31] Medical professionals must consider being responsible for their own security when entering into a disaster scenario. Law enforcement may have not had the opportunity to completely cordon off the area to protect first responders and civilians in close proximity. As described in relation to suicide attack response considerations for first responders by Forester and colleagues,[7] the first arriving units should be ready and able to begin a response for their specific agency. However, the study showed first responders are rarely prepared for, and often unaware of, the threat of secondary devices used after the initial explosion. The study also detailed how civilian response in Israel to a terrorist attack is to immediately move toward the incident to render aid, whereas in other parts of the world civilians tend to flee. This approach can be viewed as beneficial or detrimental with more personnel being in close proximity to a secondary device. If a second device detonates successfully, the effects on first responders and civilians is devastating. There are multiple examples of successful detonation of secondary devices with great success that occurred in Israel and the United States over the past 20 years. Subsequently, vigilant first responders must be aware of the threat potential and render an area safe before beginning triage and medical response to the injured.

There remains much to learn in building collective knowledge through experience from previous terrorist attacks on military personnel and international events. This process entails prior coordination between emergency services and strong communication that is established by incident command. Based on proficiency and experience, first responders tend to be aware of their surroundings and when otherwise typical circumstances seem out of place. Further educating first responders for the potential threat and warning signs of terrorist activity prompts awareness and presents a first line of defense against terrorist threats.

VEHICLE ATTACK MITIGATION AND THE ROAD AHEAD

It is evident that using vehicles as modes of terrorism to kill and injure will become more prevalent in the coming years. It is imperative that those working in defense support of civil authorities (DSCA) maintain a high level of alertness and are prepared to respond appropriately to these likely attacks. The TSA has noted that vehicular attacks are becoming more common and have warned truckers to watch for possible ramming terror attacks.[32]

Car ramming is a low-cost, less meticulous form of spreading fear that has the ability to avoid detection by law enforcement. The authorities need additional support in this regard, and paying close attention to key indicators of strange behavior is particularly important for civilians and those employed in the rental vehicle industry. The TSA has informed bus and trucking companies to pay attention to indicators, such as modifications of these automobiles, that may indicate their plan to use the vehicle for nefarious purposes. In addition, the TSA is encouraging the use of vehicle barriers or portable barriers that may help to prevent vehicles from accelerating directly into a large group of people, such as a marathon, concert, sporting event, or street market.[25] **Box 1** provides TSA guidance on potential vehicle ramming attack indicators.

The TSA has developed a set of countermeasures in partnership with public and private sector transportation security partners with the aim of aiding in preventing, protecting, and mitigating the use of commercial vehicles in terrorist attacks within the homeland.[33] These countermeasures focus on facility security and event security (on the road, rental vehicle companies, community partnership). It is highly recommended that facility programs provide vehicle accountability measures at any major event. Event security should be on high alert and should reinforce strong vehicle security,

---

Box 1
Vehicle ramming attacks: potential indicators

- Unusual and unexplained modifications to commercial motor vehicles, such as attempts to reinforce the front of the vehicle with metal plates.

- The purchase, rental, or request for temporary use of commercial motor vehicles, if accompanied by typical indicators such as nervousness during the purchase, paying in cash, or lack of familiarity with the vehicle's operations.

- Attempts by a commercial vehicle driver to unnecessarily or unlawfully infiltrate areas where crowds are gathered.

- Commercial motor vehicles being operated erratically, at unusual times, or in unusual locations, particularly in crowded pedestrian areas.

- Presentation of altered or questionable driver's license, proof of insurance, credit cards, or other required documents when purchasing or renting vehicles.

- Suspicious behavior on the part of a vehicle trainee, such as lack of interest in what type of work they will do, what route they will drive, or how much they will be paid.

From Cooper D. Vehicle Ramming Attacks (Threat Landscape, Indicators, and Countermeasures). Presentation presented at the: National Homeland Security Consortium / Transportation Security Administration (TSA). National Emergency Management Association. Available at: https://www.nemaweb.org/index.php/resources/document-library.

establish adequate vehicle standoff distance, and use vehicle barriers near parades and other celebratory gatherings, sporting events, entertainment venues, or shopping centers.[33] Rental vehicle companies are a potential source of information, and it is recommended that they report to authorities any suspicions arising from the rental of large-capacity vehicles in areas and within a proximate time frame of parades and other celebratory gatherings, sporting events, entertainment venues, shopping centers, or other activities that place crowds near roads, streets, or venues accessible by vehicles.[33] In addition, it is recommended that a request be made for increased presence and visibility of law enforcement personnel near parades and other celebratory gatherings, sporting events, entertainment venues, or shopping centers.[33]

The FBI, Department of Homeland Security, and TSA have coordinated with the Truck Renting and Leasing Association and the American Car Rental Association to aid vehicle rental employees identify suspicious activities and behaviors. Based on the indicators listed in **Box 1**, the employees should obtain a description of the individual, why the encounter was suspicious or alarming, rental agreement documents and identification documents provided by the customer, information on any associates present with the customer, and any information regarding how the customer departed the counter(ie, whether it was in a vehicle, on foot, or using public transportation).[34]

SUMMARY

Vehicle attacks present a serious terrorist threat to society that requires extreme countermeasures for mitigation and necessitates the appropriate medical response. Awareness is at the forefront of detecting and proposing plans and procedures to prevent terrorist activity. Knowledge of these types of attacks is gained through prior incidents on the battlefield and developing situational awareness of evolving tactics. It is therefore essential that civilian authorities apply lessons learned from prior vehicle attack incidents. Using Israeli tactics and medical responses to such events along with relying on the US military's evolving modus operandi in coping with such adversity will lead to reduced morbidity/mortality and hinder the terrorist goals and objectives. Medical preparedness of civilian responders in dealing with catastrophic injuries and loss of life depends on quality rehearsal and realistic training before an attack. Applying this approach offers the most prudent measure to limit the potential damage caused by vehicle attacks. Preparedness and mitigation efforts may be the best hope to weaken the terrorist movement to instill fear and remind terrorists that their efforts to coerce governments will never hinder freedom and democracy.

RESOURCES

- For more information: dhs.gov/critical-infrastructure-security
- Don't Be a Puppet: https://cve.fbi.gov
- Pathway to Violence: dhs.gov/pathway-violence-video
- Hometown Security initiative: https://www.dhs.gov/hometown-security
- If You See Something, Say Something: https://www.dhs.gov/see-something-say-something
- Nationwide Suspicious Activity Reporting Initiative: https://nsi.ncirc.gov/
- https://www.fbi.gov/video-repository/vehicle-rentals-vehicle-ramming-013019.mp4/view
- https://www.dhs.gov/sites/default/files/publications/Vehicle%20Ramming%20-%20Security%20Awareness%20for%20ST-CP.PDF

- Protective Security Advisors (PSAs) proactively engage with government partners and the private sector to protect critical infrastructure. For more information or to contact your local PSA, e-mail NICC@hq.dhs.gov

REFERENCES

1. Brobeck, B. D. (2010). Protection, Risk and Communication: Battling the Effects of Improvised Explosive Devices in Contemporary Operations. NAVAL WAR COLLEGE NEWPORT RI JOINT MILITARY OPERATIONS DEPT.
2. Bunker RJ. Daesh/IS armored vehicle borne improvised explosive devices (AV-BIEDs): insurgent use and terrorism potentials 2016. CGU Faculty Publications and Research.
3. Urwin M, Meehan N. The 1972–3 Dublin bombings. History Ireland 2018; 26(3):46–9.
4. Nesser P. Chronology of jihadism in Western Europe 1994–2007: planned, prepared, and executed terrorist attacks. Studies in Conflict & Terrorism 2008; 31(10):924–46.
5. McGuire R, Hepper A, Harrison K. From Northern Ireland to Afghanistan: half a century of blast injuries. J R Army Med Corps 2019;165(1):27–32.
6. Richman A. Patterns within nine preattack phases that emerged in Israel suicide bombing cases 2018. Walden University ScholarWorks.
7. Foerster CR, Mohr JA, Patrick JE, et al. (P2-2) Suicide Attack Response Considerations for First Responders. Prehospital and Disaster Medicine 2011;26. https://doi.org/10.1017/S1049023X11004468.
8. CEP (Counter Extremism Project). Vehicles as weapons of terror 2019. Counterextremism.com. Available at: https://www.counterextremism.com/vehicles-as-weapons-of-terror. Accessed June 7, 2019.
9. Ciottone GR, Biddinger PD, Darling RG, et al, editors. Ciottone's disaster medicine. Elsevier Health Sciences; 2015.
10. Cooper D. Vehicle Ramming Attacks (Threat Landscape, Indicators, and Countermeasures). Presentation presented at the: 2018; National Homeland Security Consortium/Transportation Security Administration (TSA).
11. Ibrahim Y. "Inspire" magazine by Al-Qaeda - CIA. 2010. Cia.gov. Available at: https://www.cia.gov/library/abbottabadcompound/81/8182F17CE93AAE7BFD4F2CB9A65E8B85_T3.DOC.pdf. Accessed June 7, 2019.
12. FBI. Terrorist use of vehicle ramming tactics. Federal Bureau of Investigation; 2010. Available at: https://info.publicintelligence.net/DHS-TerroristRamming.pdf. Accessed June 7, 2019.
13. Ladan-Baki IS, Enwere C. INTRA-ELITE CONFLICT AND PROBLEMS OF GOVERNANCE IN NIGERIA: IMPERATIVES OF GAMES THEORY IN AFRICAN POLITICS 2017.
14. Mahzam R. Rumiyah – Jihadist propaganda & information warfare in cyberspace. Counter Terrorist Trends and Analyses 2017;9(3):8–14.
15. Wilson C. Improvised explosive devices (IEDs) in Iraq and Afghanistan: effects and countermeasures. In: CRS report for congress. Washington, DC: Congressional Research Service; 2007. p. 6.
16. Wilkinson A, Bevan J, Biddle I. Improvised explosive devices (IEDs): an introduction1. In: Surplus. Small Arms Survey, Geneva: Graduate Institute of International Studies; 2008. p. 136.

17. Grant M, Stewart MG. A systems model for probabilistic risk assessment of improvised explosive device attacks. Int J Intell Defence Support Syst 2012; 5(1):75–93.

18. Mahoney P, Carr D, Harrison K, et al. Forensic reconstruction of two military combat related shooting incidents using an anatomically correct synthetic skull with a surrogate skin/soft tissue layer. International journal of legal medicine 2019; 133(1):151–62.

19. Kopp C. Technology of improvised explosive devices. Defence Today 2008; 4649:46–9.

20. Carli P, Pons F, Levraut J, et al. The French emergency medical services after the Paris and Nice terrorist attacks: what have we learnt? Lancet 2017;390(10113): 2735–8.

21. Jasiński A. Protecting public spaces against vehicular terrorist attacks. Czasopismo Techniczne 2018;2:47–56.

22. Rak L, Drozd J, Flasar Z. Selected aspects of vehicle born improvized explosive devices. In: International conference KNOWLEDGE-BASED ORGANIZATION (Vol. 23, No. 3, pp. 251–6). De Gruyter Open, June 2017.

23. Jenkins BM, Butterworth BR. Terrorist vehicle attacks on public surface transportation targets. Mineta Transportation Institute, San José State University; 2017.

24. Cancian MF. Tactics, techniques, and procedures of the Islamic state 2017. Military Review.

25. TSA. Vehicle ramming attacks (threat landscape, indicators, and countermeasures) 2017. info.publicintelligence.net. Available at: https://info.publicintelligence.net/TSA-VehicleRamming.pdf. Accessed June 7, 2019.

26. Cooper D. 2017.

27. Rahman MFA. Threats of driverless vehicles: leveraging new technologies for solutions 2016.

28. Greenberg MI, Horowitz M, Haroz R. Vehicle-borne improvised explosive devices. In: Disaster medicine. Mosby; 2006. p. 757–60.

29. Waldman M, Richman A, Shapira SC. Tactical medicine—the Israeli revised protocol. Mil Med 2012;177(1):52–5.

30. Ferreri TG, Weir AJ. EMS, improvised explosive devices and terrorist activity. In: StatPearls [Internet]. StatPearls Publishing; 2019.

31. DePalma RG, Burris DG, Champion HR, et al. Blast injuries. New England Journal of Medicine 2005;352(13):1335–42.

32. Hanna J. TSA warns truckers: watch for possible ramming terror attacks. 2017. CNN.com. Available at: http://www.cnn.com/2017/05/04/politics/tsa-ramming-terror-attacks-warning/. Accessed June 7, 2019.

33. Cooper D. 2008.

34. Sullivan M. Partners in prevention: vehicle rentals and vehicle ramming 2019. FBI.gov. Available at: https://www.fbi.gov/videorepository/vehicle-rentals-vehicle-ramming-013019.mp4/view. Accessed June 7, 2019.

Bombs and Blasts

Mary Showstark, MS, PA-C

KEYWORDS

- Bombs • Blasts • Disaster • Mass casualty • Trauma

KEY POINTS

- Bomb blasts are becoming more and more common in day-to-day life.
- Bombs can be made at home and instructions are even found on the Internet.
- In the past 15 years there has been an increase in explosives used for terrorist attacks.

INTRODUCTION

Bomb blasts are becoming more and more common in day-to-day life. Bombs can be made at home and instructions are even found on the Internet. In the past 15 years there has been an increase in explosives used for terrorist attacks. Events such as the Easter attack in Sri Lanka, the Boston Marathon, the Brussels commuter hub, and Ariana Grande concert bombings at the Manchester Arena are becoming all too common. This article considers the technical background of blast devices, describes the contextual characteristics of explosive events and their implications for response, and discusses common injuries that should not be missed in blast scenarios.

BACKGROUND

Bombs and explosives are not new technology. There have been reports of bombs being used for terrorist attacks for more than 3 decades, and there is a wide spectrum of technical means to create an explosive blast.

TYPES OF BLAST DEVICES

Improvised explosive devices (IEDs), also known as homemade devices, are created through nonindustrial means. They are usually made from civilian-use explosives, fertilizers, and repurposed military munitions. Penetrating, poisonous, and incendiary components may be added to increase lethality.

The means of delivery may also vary. IEDs were used as car and truck bombs in Oklahoma City and the first attack on the World Trade Center. In 2016, the New

Disclosure Statement: The author has nothing to disclose.
Yale School of Medicine Physician Assistant Online Program, 100 Church Street South, Suite A230, New Haven, CT 06519, USA
E-mail address: MARY.SHOWSTARK@YALE.EDU

Physician Assist Clin 4 (2019) 751–760
https://doi.org/10.1016/j.cpha.2019.06.011
2405-7991/19/© 2019 Elsevier Inc. All rights reserved.

York and New Jersey bombings, which injured more than 30 people, were carried out with an IED made from a pressure cooker.[1] The so-called Idaho Unabomber, active from 1978 to 1996, mailed IEDs to the victims in letters and packages.[2] Pipe bombs were used in the Atlanta Olympics and mailed by Cesar Sayoc from Miami to many political figures. Backpack and satchel bombs have been used in Israel and London, as well as the Boston marathon. These suitcase bombs may contain shrapnel. In 2011, the Spokane bomb contained not only shrapnel but also rat poison to prevent bleeding wounds from coagulating. Sometimes the vehicle itself may be used as an improvised bomb, such as airplanes in the 2001 World Trade Center and the Pentagon attack.

Scene

Providers may encounter blast injuries in any of these settings: from walking down the street, to attending church, to a concert event. Such large social events may easily turn into mass casualty incidents if a bomb is detonated inside the crowd. There are several important components to a successful response to an explosive mass casualty event.

Responders should have an incident command area, an area designated for multiple agencies to all be in one place. For instance, when working a marathon, there are representatives from the police, fire, ambulance, race headquarters, and other special units all in a single location. They are able to communicate with a central location to have information from the field relayed to them. The incident command area can also serve as a location to collect and gather evidence. The medical provider should be aware of what the mass casualty plan is, whether working in the prehospital or hospital environment.

The first thing that the provider must ensure is scene safety. This is among the first rules in Advanced Wilderness Life Support.[3] The area should be checked for secondary devices or suspicious packages left unattended. Things to watch out for are victims with no soft tissue injuries when everyone else appears to be injured and suspicious vehicles left unattended or leaving the scene. Either of these signs could point to the perpetrator but also could be related to secondary blast devices. The provider should also take note of locations where secondary devices could be placed, such as garbage bins and under vehicles. The provider should not jump to help people without first assessing their own safety. This includes being properly dressed. Ideally, the provider should be covered, and have eye, nose, and mask protection in the form of personal protective equipment. The provider should note that there may be shrapnel, air-borne toxins, and contaminated patients and environment, as well as dangerous patients.[4,5] Dirty bombs consist of radiological or chemical components combined with an explosive.[6] Therefore, scene safety in the prehospital setting is the first priority.

Prehospital

A provider working an incident should make sure the area is restricted so that only responders can enter. They should also not let anyone leave the scene because the person might be potential suspect and/or might be contaminated. Typically, zones are set up as hot, warm, and cold, with reference to hazmat terminology. This is related to the proximity to the epicenter of the blast. The hot zone is where most people are being treated and are likely to be contaminated. The warm zone is the area where decontamination of personnel and equipment takes place, The cold zone is the uncontaminated area where providers should be safe.[7]

After scene safety is ensured, an assessment should take place regarding the volume and the severity of casualties. The results of the assessment should be immediately transferred to a command and control center, so that required resources may be issued on time. Treatment and evacuation should also be facilitated by designation of specified treatment zones and evacuation routes. It is also very important to understand which hospitals are available for evacuation and to coordinate with them.

When these issues are settled, triage of the casualties may begin. The main goal of the triage process is to divide the patients into urgent (requiring immediate attention) and nonurgent (including the deceased). The provider should note that the injury patterns may not look like those on a typical trauma patient. Victims may have many injuries that are not visible immediately. The provider should take note of the walking wounded because, even though they are walking, they may have occult injuries. The provider should still perform triage as per a typical mass casualty protocol. They should not alter their care with regard to trauma resuscitation or transport decisions. Many patients after a blast injury, if walking, will still report to the emergency department, even after their initial triage. Providers should move through walking wounded triage quickly, asking the patient the standard neurologic questions, assessing if the patient can hear you, asking if they have pain or injuries, and making sure they stay as protected from the environment as possible. If decontamination is necessary, providers need to quickly separate and maintain these patients in the hot zone.

Many factors influence the severity of the blast injury. This can depend on the device used and whether or not the explosion occurred in an open environment, such as the targeted attacks on runners at the Boston Marathon finish line, or in a closed environment, such as the 2004 Madrid commuter train attacks in which 10 bombs exploded on 4 trains killing 191 people and injuring more than 2000 people.[8]

The distance that the person is away from the device also makes a difference because being farther away lessens the likelihood of being blown by the windblast or flying shrapnel. Victims will also be wearing varying levels of clothing that are suitable for commuting to work versus running a marathon. The severity of the resulting injuries depends on the combination of clothing type, placement, and number.

Hospital

In the hospital, providers should follow their mass casualty injury protocols. Triage is also very important, thus a designated triage officer should be appointed. The approaches to the hospital should be kept open. There is a significant chance that the hospital will be at surge capacity. It is recommended that extra providers be called in for assistance. Social workers, case managers, psychiatrists, and mental health professionals play a crucial role in assisting with the care of the blast victims and their relatives.

Blast Physics

Explosives cause the rapid conversion of a solid or liquid into a gas, resulting in a sudden release of energy. Explosives are categorized as either high-order explosives or low-order explosives (**Table 1**).[9]

Pathophysiology of Blast Injuries

There are mechanisms for the pathophysiology of blast injuries, including spalling, implosion, shearing, and irreversible work. Spalling involves shock waves moving through the tissues. Implosion is caused by gases trapped in hollow organs that compress and expand, which can cause injury such as a bowel rupture. Shearing is thought to happen when tissues are moving at different speeds creating a visceral tearing. Irreversible work refers to forces that exceed the tissue tensile strength.[4,10]

Table 1
Blast physics and types[10,11]

Types of Explosives	Shock Wave	Examples	Destruction	Incendiary Thermal Effects
High-Order Explosives	Supersonic explosion Overpressurization shock Detonate quickly	Ammonium nitrate fuel oil, TNT, C-4, nitroglycerin, dynamite	More destructive	Higher temperature and shorter time result in fireball at time of detonation
Low-Order Explosives	Subsonic explosion No overpressurization wave No detonating Release energy more slowly by deflagration (substance heated until it burns away rapidly)	Gunpowder, pipe bombs, petroleum-based bombs (eg, Molotov cocktails), or aircraft improvised as guided missiles	Less destructive	Longer thermal effect; can cause secondary fires

Data from Brahmaji Master P, Chandra Sekhar V, et al. *Blast: Pattern and Nature of Injuries.* Vol 2.; 2015. Available at: https://www.jebmh.com/data_pdf/2_Brahmaji.pdf. Accessed May 17, 2019; and Centers for Disease Control and Prevention. Explosions and Blast Injuries A Primer for Clinicians. Available at: https://www.cdc.gov/masstrauma/preparedness/primer.pdf.

Types of Injuries

Primary injuries

Primary injuries are usually caused by the blast itself. This can be due to the overpressurization wave. Typically, these are related to high-order explosives. Blunt force injuries and barotrauma are common. Primary injuries may include head, ear, and abdominal injuries. Blast lung is common owing to a pressurization buildup in the lungs, similar to a barotrauma. Ear injuries include tympanic membrane (TM) rupture and ossicle disruption.[12] Abdominal injuries may include internal bleeding and organ perforation.

Secondary injuries

Secondary injuries result from debris and bomb fragments. Secondary blast injuries are the most common cause of death because of the shrapnel wounds caused by these flying objects. These include trauma to the head, neck, chest, abdomen, and extremities. Fractures and traumatic amputations are common and soft tissue injures may occur. Providers may see only minimal external signs but should not hesitate to get a radiograph or computed tomography (CT) scan. All shrapnel wounds should be considered contaminated and proper wound washing and management should take place. During the Boston Marathon bombing, secondary blast injuries were the most common. In approximately 9 out of 43 (21%) patients who arrived at the hospital, glass, gravel, and other foreign body materials were identified.[13,14] Providers should also consider nonradiopaque debris that might not be seen in routine imaging.[13] Human remains can also become projectiles and spread infections, so vaccination status and testing for hepatitis B, hepatitis C, and human immunodeficiency virus should be considered.[13]

Tertiary injuries

Tertiary injuries can be easily missed by providers because they may involve internal bleeding, as well as contusions and abrasions. These injuries result from patients being thrown by the windblast. Head injuries, skull fractures, and bone fractures are also common.

Quaternary injuries

Injuries that are not related to primary, secondary, or tertiary mechanisms are classified as quaternary. These can be related to heat and radiation injuries. These can include burns, head injuries, and exacerbation of preexisting medical conditions, such as asthma, posttraumatic stress disorder (PTSD), high blood pressure, chest pain, and anxiety.

Crush injuries can also be classified as quaternary. Crush injuries occur when a body part is placed under a high degree of pressure, that is, crushed for a prolonged period of time. Patients may be pinned under a car or a collapsed building. Ischemia may occur, as well as fractures. These patients should be monitored for compartment syndrome.

Compartment syndrome is a sequela of crush injuries. The affected area does not perfuse and the pressure builds up inside that area. This compromises circulation and the function of the area affected. If structural collapse is involved, several questions need to be asked: Are there victims who need to be rescued? If they did escape, how long were they stuck under prolonged pressure? The provider should remember the 5 Ps from physical examination: pain, pallor, paresthesia, paralysis, and pulselessness. The affected area should be immobilized. The provider should be mindful of compartment syndrome and monitor compartment pressures and the need for a fasciotomy of the affected area. Ideally, the fasciotomy is performed by a surgeon;

however, there is a guide for the direction in which a fasciotomy should be performed (http://www.wheelessonline.com/ortho/12806).[15,16]

Providers should also watch for crush syndrome. Crush syndrome is anything related to the crush injury, including compartment syndrome, but it may occur in the absence of trauma. Reasons include a possible deep venous thrombosis, anemia, toxins, preexisting medication, or drugs of abuse. Rhabdomyolysis and reperfusion injury may occur with these patients. Patients my present dehydrated or in shock, or with mental status changes or hypothermia or hyperthermia.[10]

Providers should monitor electrolytes and kidney function and watch for metabolic acidosis and acute renal failure. These patients should be given aggressive fluid resuscitation but also diuretics. Dialysis may be needed.[4] The provider should maintain a balance because they do not want to create compartment syndrome; however, this may be unavoidable. These patients should receive aggressive pain control.

Combined injuries

Combined injuries are sometimes known as quinary injuries. Here the provider can see a combination of multiple injuries. It should be noted that providers in the field or in the surge that enters the hospital may feel overwhelmed. Providers should not just focus in on a distracting injury. Patients may have burns or blast lung, as well as globe rupture or traumatic brain injury (TBI). Providers should take a step back and remember their advanced life support training and concentrate on airway, breathing, and circulation. Providers should also note that patients may have burns or crush injuries, and remember not to overload these patients with fluid due to the risk of development of pulmonary edema and compartment syndrome (**Tables 2 and 3**).

Blast Lung

Blast lung, as previously mentioned, occurs when the patient's lungs have an over-pressurization. Think of the lungs as 2 balloons; in these chambers the pressure is building up, increasing intrathoracic pressure. Anything inside the lung becomes susceptible to intense pressure. This can lead to alveolar tearing, hemorrhage, edema, and possible rupture. Pulmonary contusion, pneumothorax, hemothorax, pneumomediastinum, and subcutaneous emphysema may be found. Providers should look for symptoms such as hypoxia, wheezing, cyanosis, tachypnea, decreased breath sounds, respiratory distress, and bloody sputum.[4,9,10,14] Providers should use their stethoscopes and their physical examination skills to check for fremitus and percussion, especially when in the field, in order to not miss these patients. Chest radiograph

Table 2				
Frequency of bomb blast cases during the period from 2007 to 2011 at Karachi				
Year	Blasts	Persons Dead	Persons Injured	Total
2007	3	85	260	345
2008	1	08	26	34
2009	2	43	77	120
2010	9	65	371	436
2011	31	48	159	207
Total	46	249	893	1142

From Mirza FH, Parhyar HA, Tirmizi SZ. Rising threat of terrorist bomb blasts in Karachi–a 5-year study. J Forensic Leg Med. 2013 Aug;20(6):747-51. https://doi.org/10.1016/j.jflm.2013.04.014. Epub 2013 May 29; with permission.

Table 3
Frequency of cause of death in bomb blast victims

Cause of Death	Number of Cases	Percentage (%)
Head injury with or without hemorrhage	37	14.86
Injury of chest and abdomen with or without head injury	30	12.05
Shock due to multiple injuries	156	62.65
Chronic renal failure due to shock and injuries	14	5.62
Fragmented body remains (shattering)	12	4.82
Total	249	100

From Mirza FH, Parhyar HA, Tirmizi SZ. Rising threat of terrorist bomb blasts in Karachi–a 5-year study. J Forensic Leg Med. 2013 Aug;20(6):747-51. https://doi.org/10.1016/j.jflm.2013.04.014. Epub 2013 May 29; with permission.

may show pulmonary infiltrates or contusions with a butterfly-like pattern. Bilateral hilar pulmonary edema also may be seen on radiograph. Arterial blood gas testing is also useful in the management of these patients. Air emboli, such as acute gas embolism, should be considered if a rapid decline in mental status occurs.[9] There is a debate about whether or not blast lung appears within 2 hours of the blast or can appear up to 48 hours later.[17]

Treatment of blast lung includes high-flow oxygen, nonrebreather mask, and continuous positive airway pressure. Intubation may be imminent for these patients. Providers should not overload these patients with fluids and should treat them similar to patients with pulmonary contusions. There is a blast lung severity score that looks at the ratio of Pao_2 to fraction of inspired oxygen (Fio_2), chest radiograph findings, and the presence of bronchopleural fistula.[10]

Head Injuries

Primary blast waves can cause concussion or mild TBI. This can occur without a direct blow to the head. Patients may have a TBI such as intracranial hemorrhage, which may be a subdural, subarachnoid, or cerebral contusion. Diffuse axonal injury may also be seen. The blast itself can cause such pressure inside the human head cavity it can affect all areas of the brain. Providers should note if patients are complaining of headaches, are confused, or having balance issues. The victim may have trouble hearing. All of these symptoms should be looked at and watched because these could be symptoms of a mild TBI. Victims may complain of being tired or weak, be unable to focus, be unable to remember what exactly happened, or lose consciousness. The provider should monitor these patients to see if this is a concussion or elements of PTSD.

CT scan imaging of the head and cervical spine should be obtained on these patients. Remember that penetrating trauma may still be present from shrapnel even though the patient does not look injured externally. Cervical spine injuries can be present and the spine should be immobilized in a collar until the patient can be cleared. All head injury patients should be observed because ventilatory support may be needed. Neurosurgical consults are also useful. Close attention to those TBI patients who require intubation or who have decompensated should include cerebral perfusion pressure, sedation, seizure prophylaxis, monitoring of glucose, and temperature control.[9]

Ears and Eye Injuries

Tympanic membrane ruptures are very common in blast injuries. Hearing loss or TM rupture has an apparent association with the quantity of the explosion and the distance from the explosion.[12] Tympanic membrane rupture may be found alone or with a combination of injuries. Ossicular disruption, cochlear damage, and middle ear damage may occur. In the field, these patients may not be able to hear the provider. The provider may think that the patient is acting bizarrely and may have a TBI, or is ignoring them. Providers should try to approach these patients from the side, ensure that they are seated, and not stand over them. Providers should attempt empathetic gestures such as placing their hand on the victim's shoulder or gently stroking the patient's arm to let them know that they are there trying to take care of them. Some patients may complain solely of tinnitus, which will resolve in time.

Patients suffering from blast injuries to the ear may have conductive or sensorineural hearing loss. Weber and Rinne tests can be performed for a quick analysis. Providers should note blood in the external ear canal. On otoscopic examination, providers may find debris or foreign bodies in the canal, TM rupture, cochlear damage, or ossicular disruption.

Usually, the TM heals on its own. If sensorineural hearing loss is present, this is typically permanent and the provider will need to explain this to the patient. Ear, nose, and throat specialist consultation and audiometry are needed for these patients.

Eye injuries can entail retinitis, hyphema, globe injuries, and possible rupture. Corneal burns, retinal detachments, and corneal lacerations may be present. Patients may complain of foreign body sensation, pain, irritation, and vision changes. Providers might note apparent debris, erythema, vision loss, or note periorbital swelling. Patients should be referred to an ophthalmologist immediately.

Abdominal Injuries

Abdominal injuries are sometimes referred to as blast abdomen. The internal hollow organs perforate and the solid organs have the potential to lacerate. Patients with gastrointestinal symptoms postblast should be evaluated. Patients may experience abdominal pain, nausea, vomiting blood, or rectal or testicular pain. Patients may present as hypotensive. Providers should check the abdomen by first inspecting; auscultating, because bowel signs may be absent; and percussing. Next, they should use light and deep palpation to check for any peritoneal signs such as rebound and guarding. The colon is the most common location for perforation and hemorrhage. Testicular rupture can also occur.

Providers should not hesitate to get plain films and CT scan, which may show penetrating foreign bodies and free air. Retroperitoneal and mesenteric injuries may also be present.

Special Considerations

Special considerations should be taken for pregnant women, children, the elderly, and disabled persons.

Pregnant women should remain in the hospital for fetal monitoring because there is a risk of placenta detachment. Pelvic ultrasounds and fetal nonstress test-monitoring should be performed, and an obstetrician-gynecologist should be immediately consulted.

Children are at a greater risk for blast lung. Often, children seem quite resilient in trauma situations; however, the provider must remember that, even though the child may be walking and talking, they can decompensate quickly.

The elderly are another subset of the special populations. They are at risk for increased hospital stays, intensive care unit admissions, and orthopedic fractures due to decreased bone density.

Patients with walkers and wheelchairs may need their devices decontaminated. Providers should note that patients who are not able to answer may have suffered a

TM rupture, be scared, or speak another language; or are hard of hearing, deaf, or deaf and blind. Providers must remember to consult appropriate specialists, including pediatricians, social workers, translators, and case managers.[4,9]

Mental Health

After a blast, as previously discussed, the potential for a TBI is quite possible. According to recent literature, TBI and psychiatric issues such as anxiety, depression, and PTSD may occur (**Appendix 1**).[18] PTSD with postconcussive syndrome is also known to occur.

Many patients will be understandably distraught after coming in contact with a blast injury. Many military professionals can suffer from PTSD. This can also affect civilians who encounter such incidents. In 2012, a study based in Tanzania looked at children who had been exposed to bombs that were stockpiled in Mbagala, Dar es Salaam. Stockpiled military bombs exploded, injuring approximately 600 people and destroying 9049 homes. The study compared children exposed to the bombs and those from a nearby town and found that 93% of children experienced PTSD, with no differences noted for gender.[19]

SUMMARY

In this changing environment, medical providers may come into contact with bomb and blast injuries. They must understand that there are different types of explosives with different resultant injuries and these may vary in closed and open environments. These injuries may not be apparent initially; however, providers should familiarize themselves with appropriate mass casualty protocols and triage.

Injuries may be classified from primary to quaternary, including combined injuries (quinary). Providers should always rely on their physical examination skills and be liberal with imaging. Mental health sequelae must be taken into consideration (see **Appendix 1**).

REFERENCES

1. How the bomb Squad disabled a Second explosive in the Chelsea bombing - the New York times. Available at: https://www.nytimes.com/2017/10/05/nyregion/chelsea-bombing-trial.html. Accessed May 17, 2019.
2. Unabomber — FBI. Available at: https://www.fbi.gov/history/famous-cases/unabomber. Accessed May 17, 2019.
3. Auerbach PS. Advanced wilderness life support: prevention, diagnosis, treatment, evacuation. Wilderness Medicine Society; 2011.
4. Bombings. Available at: https://www.acep.org/globalassets/uploads/...files/.../cdc.../bombings3h.ppt. Accessed May 17, 2019.
5. Blast Event universal blast scene safety bombings: injury patterns and care pocket guide secondary, tertiary, and quaternary injuries are common in blast events, and large majority are not critical. It is unlikely to experience patients with injuries isolated to one category. A more likely scenario would be to experience patients with a combination of all the injuries listed below. Treatment for most of these blast injuries follows established protocols for that specific injury. Primary injuries. Available at: www.bt.cdc.gov/masscasualties/. Accessed May 17, 2019.
6. Backgrounder on dirty bombs. Available at: https://www.nrc.gov/reading-rm/doc-collections/fact-sheets/fs-dirty-bombs.html. Accessed May 17, 2019.
7. US EPA O. Safety Zones. Available at: https://www.epa.gov/emergency-response/safety-zones. Accessed May 17, 2019.

8. Terrorists bomb trains in Madrid - HISTORY. Available at: https://www.history.com/this-day-in-history/terrorists-bomb-trains-in-madrid. Accessed May 17, 2019.

9. Bombings and blast injuries: a primer for Physicians. Available at: https://www.aapsus.org/wp-content/uploads/ajcmfour.pdf. Accessed May 17, 2019.

10. Brahmaji Master P, Chandra Sekhar V, Rangaiah YKC, et al. Blast: pattern and nature of injuries, vol. 2, 2015. Available at: https://www.jebmh.com/data_pdf/2_Brahmaji.pdf. Accessed May 17, 2019.

11. Explosions and blast injuries a primer for Clinicians.

12. Effects of bomb blast injury on the ears: the Aga Khan University Hospital experience. Available at: https://advance.lexis.com/document/?pdmfid=1516831&crid=3d8d05be-6804-48fc-b757-5a08175605ed&pddocfullpath=%2Fshared%2Fdocument%2Fnews%2Furn%3AcontentItem%3A5PJS-NSC1-F00C-62FR-00000-00&pddocid=urn%3AcontentItem%3A5PJS-NSC1-F00C-62FR-00000-00&pdcontentcom. Accessed May 17, 2019.

13. Brunner J, Singh AK, Rocha T, et al. Terrorist bombings: foreign bodies from the boston marathon bombing. Semin Ultrasound CT MR 2015;36(1):68–72.

14. Gates JD, Arabian S, Biddinger P, et al. The initial response to the boston marathon bombing. Ann Surg 2014;260(6):960–6.

15. Wheeless' Textbook of Orthopaedics. Available at: http://www.wheelessonline.com/ortho/12806. Accessed May 27, 2019.

16. Masquelet A-C. Acute compartment syndrome of the leg: pressure measurement and fasciotomy. Orthop Traumatol Surg Res 2010;96(8):913–7.

17. Hare SS, Goddard I, Ward P, et al. The radiological management of bomb blast injury. Clin Radiol 2007;62(1):1–9.

18. American Psychiatric Association. Diagnostic and statistical manual of mental disorders, fifth Edition (DSM-5). Arlington (TX): American Psychiatric Association; 2013. p. 2013.

19. Messo IN. Prevalence of post-traumatic stress disorder in children: the case of the Mbagala bomb blasts in Tanzania. J Health Psychol 2013;18(5):627–37. https://doi.org/10.1177/1359105312451188.

APPENDIX

Appendix 1
PTSD Summary of Diagnostic and Statistical Manual of Mental Disorders, 5th edition, Criteria
Subjected to real or threatened death or grave physical harm either by experiencing, witnessing, learning about it, or exposure to repeated details (providers encounter the latter)
Intruding symptoms, such as difficult memories, dreams, flashbacks, marked physiologic reactions that symbolize the traumatic event (1 or more)
Circumvention of the event, memories, feelings, people, situations
Variance in mood and cognition: feeling as if it is their fault; dissociation with the event; blame, horror, anger, guilt, or shame; unable to feel positive emotions; inability to remember the event (2 or more)
Noticeable variation in stimulation: hypervigilance, irritability, anger, outbursts, recklessness, problems with concentration, sleep disturbances (2 or more)
Duration of the previous categorizations greater than 1 month
Disturbances cause significant strain in work or home environment
Disturbances are not related to other medical conditions

Data from American Psychiatric Association. Diagnostic and Statistical Manual of Mental Disorders, Fifth Edition (DSM-5), American Psychiatric Association, Arlington 2013.; 2013.

Mass Shootings and Health Care: An Epidemic?

Mary Showstark, MS, PA-C

KEYWORDS

- Active shooter • Health care • Mass shootings • Mental health

KEY POINTS

- There is no typical profile for an active shooter.
- Providers should look out for patients who are depressed and feel bullied.
- Asking specific questions that focus on the psychiatric review of systems and social history are key elements to helping find out if a patient may be at risk of becoming an active shooter.

INTRODUCTION

Mass shootings, also known as mass killings, and active shooter incidents are all too common. Mass shootings are defined by the Congressional Research Service as events where more than 4 people within one event or in close proximity are killed with a firearm. Congress uses the term mass killings and defines this as 3 or more killings in a single incident. The Federal Bureau of Investigations (FBI) uses the term active shooter, which is an individual who is trying to actively kill or attempt to kill people in a crowded area.[1] As of mid-May 2019, there have been 137 mass shootings.[2] In 2018 there were 27 shootings in which 85 people were killed and 128 people wounded.[3] From 2000 to 2017 there were 250 active shooter incidents in the United States[4] (**Fig. 1**). This epidemic is not going away. The active shooter is something that the provider needs to be aware of. This article aims to inform the provider of the background of mass shootings, what things to look for, how to interact if in a situation with an active shooter, and resources to plan and provide care for victims.

BACKGROUND

The Second Amendment guarantees an individual right to bear arms specifically stating, "A well-regulated Militia, being necessary to the security of a free State, the right of the people to keep and bear Arms, shall not be infringed." This amendment is continuously argued.[5] Was the point for everyone to bear arms? What does a regulated militia exactly

Yale School of Medicine Physician Assistant Online Program, 100 Church Street South, Suite A230, New Haven, CT 06519, USA
E-mail address: MARY.SHOWSTARK@YALE.EDU

Physician Assist Clin 4 (2019) 761–779
https://doi.org/10.1016/j.cpha.2019.06.006
2405-7991/19/© 2019 Elsevier Inc. All rights reserved.

physicianassistant.theclinics.com

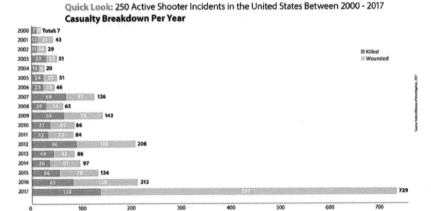

Fig. 1. Active shooter incidents in the United States between 2000 and 2017. (*From* Quick Look: 250 Active Shooter Incidents in the United States Between 2000-2017 — FBI. https://www.fbi.gov/about/partnerships/office-of-partner-engagement/active-shooter-incidents-graphics. Accessed May 23, 2019.)

mean? One will never know the true intention of the amendment written during the Philadelphia Convention, also known as the Constitutional Convention in 1787. The fact of the matter is, guns are around and available and we need to look at how to minimize and stop active shooters by analyzing the events and preattack behaviors.

A study of preattack behaviors conducted by the FBI states that shooters are mostly men. Studies examining 63 active shooting incidents between 2000 and 2013 and another in 2018 found that 94% were men, single (57%) or divorced or separated (22%), and mostly white (63%),[6] although the FBI states that violence is gender neutral and threats made by women should not be seen as just "fantasy or attention-seeking behavior."[7]

A study conducted by the US Secret Service and US Department of Education in 2004 found that in school shootings the acts were never random attacks. Before the attack other people may have known about the attacker's idea and/or plans; however, persons were not typically threatened directly. There were no set demographic or traits to "profile" the attacker. Most attackers demonstrated behaviors before that possibly indicated a need for help, some had even considered or attempted suicide. Many attackers felt bullied or injured by others and many of them had used weapons before attack. Many student attackers did not have a diagnosis of a mental disorder, although some had a history of depressive signs and suicidal attempts.[8]

Threat assessment is real and many providers may not recognize that this is part of their job. Although governmental profiling is not a skill a provider is taught, the abovementioned studies show that a typical "profile" does not fully exist. Clinicians should remain astute to their patients, because many of the abovementioned signs and symptoms could be elicited in their clinical interview. Providers should not hesitate to report that people (maybe state patients and/or people) they suspect that demonstrate behaviors they find concerning (**Fig. 2**). They should ask patients if they feel bullied. Providers oftentimes become busy and hesitate to ask social history questions or psychiatric review of systems. We have to remember that we may be the first people involved in a future active shooter's care. Providers need to be diligent with questions and recognize signs and symptoms that may lead to violence.

It is noted that violence can be characterized in two ways which are predatory/planned or impulsive/reactive. The first way is how it sounds; the act is premeditated. The latter is frequently emotional and not thought out, occasionally in response to a

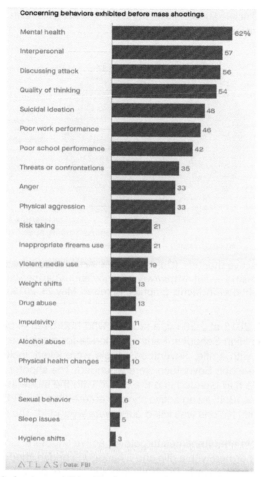

Concerning behaviors exhibited before mass shootings

Mental health	62%
Interpersonal	57
Discussing attack	56
Quality of thinking	54
Suicidal ideation	48
Poor work performance	46
Poor school performance	42
Threats or confrontations	35
Anger	33
Physical aggression	33
Risk taking	21
Inappropriate firearms use	21
Violent media use	19
Weight shifts	13
Drug abuse	13
Impulsivity	11
Alcohol abuse	10
Physical health changes	10
Other	8
Sexual behavior	6
Sleep issues	5
Hygiene shifts	3

ATLAS Data: FBI

Fig. 2. Concerning behaviors exhibited before mass shootings. (*From* Timmons, H. The FBI's warning signs of a mass shooter. *Quartz.* 13 November 2018. Available at: https://qz.com/1456558/the-fbis-warning-signs-of-a-mass-shooter/. Accessed May 24, 2019.)

perceived threat. Mass shootings are targeted mass attacks. They are thought out. They take planning and forethought. This is not a spontaneous act. Many people will say that active shooters just snapped but this is a misnomer. These acts are planned.[7] These acts can occur in several different settings including commerce, open space, education, government, residences, houses of worship, health care facilities, and other locations[4] (**Fig. 3**). Providers need to note that they might not only be taking care of victims of an active shooter; they too may be in the path of the killer.

MASS SHOOTING EVENTS

In a study by the FBI between 2000 and 2013, 160 active shooter incidents were analyzed and noted that the victims had no specific similarities. There was no specific age, gender, ethnicity, religion, or race noted. During the first 7 years of the study an average of 6.4 incidents occurred annually. In the last 7 years of the studies, the average increased to 16.4 annually. On average the attacks only lasted minutes; however, the emotional stress can last a lifetime.

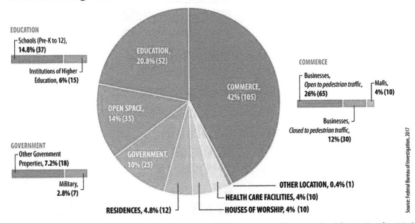

Quick Look: 250 Active Shooter Incidents in the United States From 2000 to 2017
Location Categories

Fig. 3. Locations of active shooters. (Quick Look: 250 Active Shooter Incidents in the United States Between 2000-2017 — FBI. https://www.fbi.gov/about/partnerships/office-of-partner-engagement/active-shooter-incidents-graphics. Accessed May 23, 2019.)

On February 14, 2018 at 2:30 PM, a student who had been expelled from Marjory Stoneman Douglas High School in Parkland, Florida for disciplinary reasons entered the school, armed with a rifle. Seventeen people were killed, including 14 students, 2 coaches, and 1 teacher. Seventeen were wounded. The shooter was apprehended 75 minutes later. He had blended into the crowd with the students evacuating.

On April 3, 2018 at 12:45 PM an active shooter entered the YouTube Headquarters in San Bruno, California. No one was killed but 4 were wounded. The shooter committed suicide.

Houses of Worship are oftentimes targets for active shooters. On October 27, 2018 at 9:45 AM a shooter armed with a rifle and 3 handguns began shooting inside the Tree of Life Synagogue in Pittsburgh, Pennsylvania. Eleven people were killed and 6 were wounded. The shooter was apprehended.

On November 2, 2018 at 5:37 PM, an active shooter walked into a space where one would never assume to be a victim, Hot Yoga in Tallahassee, Florida. Two people were killed and 5 were wounded. The shooter committed suicide.

Helen Vine Recovery Center, a health care facility in San Rafael, California was a target on November 5th, 2018 at 1:30 AM, and Mercy Hospital and Medical Center in Chicago, Illinois fell victim to an active shooter. The shooter shot his former fiancé, an emergency room doctor in the parking lot, then shot 2 people inside the hospital. The shooter committed suicide after being shot by law enforcement (**Table 1**).

MENTAL HEALTH

Active shooters typically target their locations. No location is safe. Providers should recognize warning signs and ask questions about the patient's home environment, feelings of depression and anxiety, safety, feeling bullied, suicidal, and homicidal ideations, noting if they have any type of plan and assessing for schizophrenia-hearing voices, sounds, or other abnormal stimuli. They should also ask if patients have a gun at home or access to one. However, are you actually allowed to ask your patients if they have a gun? Florida in 2011 had a bill placed by Governor Rick Scott that

Table 1				
Mass shootings in the United States 2002–2019				
Shootings	**Year**	**City, State**	**Killed**	**Wounded**
El AL Israeli Airlines ticket counter, LAX international Airport	July 4th, 2002	Los Angeles, California	2	2
Virginia Tech	2007	Blacksburg, Virginia	32	17
Target	2007	Kansas City, Missouri	2	8
LA Fitness Gym	2009	Collier Township, Pennsylvania	3	9
Fort Hood Soldier Retreat	2009	Fort Hood, Texas	13	32
Aurora Movie Theater	2012	Aurora, Colorado	12	58
Sandy Hook Elementary School	2012	Newton, Connecticut	27 including mother prior	2
Planned Parenthood	2015	Colorado Springs, Colorado	3	9
Pulse Nightclub[9]	2016	Orlando, Florida	49	53
Ft Lauderdale Airport	2017	Ft. Lauderdale, Florida	5	8
Bronx-Lebanon Hospital Center	2017	Bronx, New York	1	6
Route 91 Harvest Festival	2017	Las Vegas, Nevada	58	489
First Baptist Church	2017	Sutherland, Texas	26	20
Torrance Bowling Alley	2019	Torrance, California	3	4
STEM School Highlands Ranch Shooting	2019	Highlands Ranch, Colorado	1	8
University of North Carolina	2019	Charlotte, North Carolina	2	4
Memorial Day Weekend Family Barbecue	2019	Chesapeake, Virginia	1	9

Data from Refs.[3,9–12]

basically stated providers should not ask people whether or not they have a gun unless the provider believes that the safety of the patient or others is at risk. It also states that providers should not discriminate if their patients own firearms. This goes for mental health providers as well. The law even states that the question should not be on an intake form (https://www.myfloridahouse.gov/Sections/Documents/loaddoc.aspx?FileName=h0155z.JDC.DOCX&DocumentType=Analysis&BillNumber=0155&Session=2011).

Penalties include facing fines up to 10,000 dollars or loss of a medical license if this is violated. Gabrielle Gifford who is an American politician from Arizona was shot in the head with a Glock pistol in an active shooter incident. The shooter shot 24 others, killing 6 and wounding 18. Gifford spoke out against this law in a campaign "Docs versus Glocks." Although the law does not make it illegal for providers to ask, many, including Gifford, state that providers are now hesitant to ask such questions for fear of fines or losing their license. Providers should see if other such laws exist in their states but should still be diligent and document their concerns in order to justify the questions being asked.[13–15]

There is a stigma in the news that people with mental illness can be dangerous people. The reality is only 3% to 5% of violent acts are committed by people with mental illness; however, this is not said if people have not been diagnosed and approximately 3 million people with mental health issues are not receiving care. There is also claim that poverty can exacerbate behavioral problems and reducing aggressive behaviors is most effective in children versus later in life.[16] Some lay claim that inequality and income combined can be strongly associated with mass shootings.[17] The U.S. Secret Service, in 2018, found that 2/3rd of the attackers had mental health issues, almost all made threats or had concerning communications before the attacks occurred, and most had "at least one significant stressor" happen in the five years prior to the attack. There has been a noticeable increase in mental health issues in recent years; however, it is unclear as to whether or not more individuals are now seeking help.[18]

In reports upward of 60% of active shooters displayed acute paranoia, delusions, and depressive symptoms. In the Aurora, Colorado shooting, James Holmes was seeing a psychiatrist specializing in schizophrenia; Jared Loughner made classmates feel unsafe and would laugh randomly right before he shot Congresswoman Gifford. Adam Lanza, the active shooter in an elementary school in Newtown, CT, wrote stories of killings and psychologists speculate if he was an undiagnosed schizophrenic.[19,20] As providers we need to look for a combination of signs and symptoms. Mental illness alone does not cause gun violence.[21]

Nikolas Cruz, the shooter at Marjory Stoneman Douglas High School in Florida was expelled for possibly carrying a firearm onto school property. He had posts on YouTube stating he was going to become a professional school shooter. Law enforcement had 45 calls within 10 years of erratic behavior, violence, and elder abuse. He was never referred for mental health, although his lawyers argue otherwise, stating he was at one point referred, however, nothing was documented, and thus was able to legally obtain 10 guns including assault rifles.

The Brady Handgun Violence Prevention Act created in response to the assignation attempt on President Ronal Reagan requires individuals to go through a background check. These checks are conducted by the FBI's National Instant Criminal Background Check System (NICS), although some states are allowing state or local review. The NICS check is to prohibit firearms to those with prior jail time more than a year, domestic violence convictions, restraining orders, addiction, suicide attempts, and severe mental illness.[21,22] The Obama administration had required the social security administration to disclose to NICS who was on disability for a mental illness; however, in 2017 that was redacted due to multiple oppositions. NICS relies on states to submit mental health records. US Department of Justice found New Jersey and Pennsylvania uploaded more than one million records in 2015 but Alaska, Montana, Oklahoma, and other states uploaded fewer than 110. Seung-Hui Cho, the Virginia Tech killer, would have been stopped had Virginia submitted the records.[22]

Providers in no way are 100% responsible for whether or not their patient becomes an active shooter; however, providers can ask patients how they felt when witnessing a shooting or what they felt about recent news briefs they saw if not affected. This can be helpful to assess not only the patient's current mind set noting if they are experiencing any posttraumatic stress or whether or not they seem overly intrigued and at risk for violent behavior. Questions arise whether or not this "copycat" effect also known as a contagion effect is a possibility. Studies of the contagion effect cite evidence of contagion specifically with school shootings and these can be contagious for an average of 13 days.[23] Questions arise whether or not the media could portray the killers as cowards or present only the facts and not describe extensive detail. This could lead to others obtaining an excitement from this although media exposure is controversial.[18] In others affected it could lead to more stressors.[24] Threats of school violence clustering post-Columbine shootings suggested that this was a form of imitation. Providers need to check in with their patients what they are potentially concerned about, with regard to their emotional state and how they are being affected. Timing can play a pivotal role.

With regard to timing, one study looked at 3 years of data from 2013 to 2015 on mass shootings to analyze a seasonal occurrence and it was found more occurred in the summer, peak beginning in May and finishes around September to October.[25] Could this be a time where more providers check in with their patients?

The provider may be the first to encounter an active shooter in an office visit, may be the first on the scene, or may see the victims in the hospital; however, one thing providers must be very vigilant of is patients who have been victims of these attacks and their mental well-being.

It is known that persons who witness or who are around mass shootings experience depression, anxiety, and posttraumatic stress-like symptoms, which all may develop into posttraumatic stress disorder (PTSD), major depression, and generalized anxiety disorder. Psychological effects may affect family and friends of those injured as well as affect first responders, hospital staff, and the surrounding community known as vicarious trauma. Emergency responders have twice the risk of developing PTSD.[26] One-third of people involved either as direct victims, their families, or the first responders are likely to develop posttraumatic stress disorder due to being near or exposed to the trauma, which is also known as, vicarious trauma. Among those who develop PTSD, one-third of them fail to recover after 10 years.[27]

Two students from Marjorie Stoneman Douglas were found dead approximately 1 year later and 2 students separately committed suicide within a week of each other. Many speculate survivor guilt, which was discussed in interviews with students from Virginia Tech approximately 10 years later, where many students discussed their feelings of guilt, depression, anxiety, and questions of whether or not they were actually a victim or not because they survived.[28]

In 1999, thirteen people were killed and more than 20 others wounded in Columbine High School in Littleton, Colorado. In May 2019, Columbine Survivor who witnessed his best friend's death was found dead. In the years postshooting, he struggled with addiction, arrests, a failed marriage, and estrangement from his family. No cause of death has been identified and consequences are only speculated to be related to the incident.

A fascinating public health initiative, postshooting, community response occurred outside of the United States in Norway where 2 coordinated terrorist attacks occurred, one bombing in Oslo and the other in Utøya Island. The attack on the island was at a Norwegian Labor Party summer camp performed by someone who opposed the Party's views. The shooter dressed in a police officer's uniform killed 69 and injured 110. The outreach strategy postincident involved multiple crisis teams, which made constant contact with those hospitalized, nonadmitted, families and bereaved families. Each person affected was assigned a point of contact handler from Norway's public health system who monitored their mental health. They used a scale based off the UCLA PTSD Reaction index with additional questions. They noted for sleep disturbances and social isolation. The United States does not currently have a model like this in place; however, US Public Health Services as well as public health educational institutions are working on creating resources.[26]

Another long-term sequela is lead toxicity due to retained bullet fragments (RBF). From 2003 to 2012, data from the Center for Disease Control (CDC) shows approximately 457 adult shooting survivors tested positive for elevated blood levels from RBF. The CDC has a program known as Adult Blood Lead Epidemiology and Surveillance, which was present in 41 states up until 2013, which requires laboratories and providers to report blood levels to the state health departments.[29] This is particularly important for providers to ask their patients if they have RBF. In most situations, trauma surgeons leave in bullets, as the risk of going "digging" for them can actually make the situation worse; however, as years pass fragments are dissolving into the blood stream.

Colin Goddard who was shot at Virginia Tech discussed how he felt he was past the shooting and survived but now finds out that the fatigue he had been suffering from was due to elevated lead levels in his body. Lead levels can lead to neurologic problems and kidney and reproductive issues. Symptoms of elevated lead levels can be as vague as fatigue, abdominal pain, and memory loss. In an article in Time Magazine, Goddard was quoted that he was told the following: "You're going to be fine in the long-term,' and that's not right…It throws you back when you realize you're not out of the woods yet, and this terrible day is not entirely behind you."[30] Victims believe that they are now suffering again not only physically but also mentally. Providers need to ensure they ask about RBF in all of their patients and test blood lead levels when appropriate. Providers should ask about RBF when assessing past medical history, just as if asking about hypertension or diabetes as well as assessing a psychiatric review of systems at the minimum with every patient.

Medical providers need to not only work to ensure that they work through their own stressors related to vicarious trauma but also help the medical response of the people and community to increase resilience.[27,31] Some literature puts the onus on mental health providers and providers to report and hold them accountable.[19] Educators are also being encouraged to report. But is this legal, what are the rules with regard to patient-protected information and educational privacy (**Table 2**)?

THE HEALTH INSURANCE PORTABILITY AND ACCOUNTABILITY ACT OF 1996 AND THE FAMILY EDUCATIONAL RIGHTS AND PRIVACY ACT

Providers and educators are covered under HIPPA and FERPA when reporting.

Table 2		
HIPPA and FERPA during an active shooter incident		
Law	**Brief Definition of Law**	**Exceptions to Rules with Regard to Law Enforcement**
The Health Insurance Portability and Accountability Act of 1996 (HIPAA) Privacy Rule	Provides Federal privacy protections for individually identifiable health information, called protected health information or PHI, held by most health care providers and health plans and their business associates.	• To report PHI to a law enforcement official reasonably able to prevent or lessen a serious and imminent threat to the health or safety of an individual or the public. • To report PHI that the covered entity in good faith believes to be evidence of a crime that occurred on the premises. • To alert law enforcement to the death of the individual, when there is a suspicion that death resulted from criminal conduct. • When responding to an off-site medical emergency, as necessary to alert law enforcement to criminal activity.

(continued on next page)

Table 2 (*continued*)		
Law	**Brief Definition of Law**	**Exceptions to Rules with Regard to Law Enforcement**
		• To report PHI to law enforcement when required by law to do so (such as reporting gunshots or stab wounds). • To comply with a court order or court-ordered warrant, a subpoena or summons issued by a judicial officer, or an administrative request from a law enforcement official (the administrative request must include a written statement that the information requested is relevant and material, specific and limited in scope, and deidentified information cannot be used). • To respond to a request for PHI for purposes of identifying or locating a suspect, fugitive, material witness, or missing person, but the information must be limited to basic demographic and health information about the person.
The Family Educational Rights and Privacy Act (FERPA)	Law that protects the privacy of student education records. Generally, schools may disclose personally identifiable information (PII) from students' education records to outside parties, including local law enforcement, only if the parent or the eligible student has provided prior written consent.	• Schools may nonconsensually disclose designated "directory information" to law enforcement agencies. • Schools may nonconsensually disclose PII from education records in connection with a health or safety emergency. • Schools may nonconsensually disclose PII from education records in order to comply with a judicial order or a lawfully issued subpoena.

Data from HIPAA Guidance — FBI. https://www.fbi.gov/file-repository/hipaa-guide.pdf/view. Accessed May 23, 2019; and FERPA Guidance — FBI. https://www.fbi.gov/file-repository/ferpa-guide.pdf/view. Accessed May 23, 2019.

WHAT TO DO IF AN ACTIVE SHOOTER IS WHERE YOU ARE

There are a few plans that the FBI and the Health care and Public Health Sector Coordinating Council recommend if an active shooter is where you are. They essentially all cover the same thing which is, for those who are in the line of fire, to have a plan. One such plan is the Run, Hide, Fight Active Shooter Response Plan. Here, when one hears gunshots, one should run, hide, and fight if necessary. One should always try to escape and evacuate and encourage others to leave with them. One should not let others slow them down. It is recommended to remember to leave all personal belongings behind. The goal is trying to get oneself out of harm's way and out of the line of fire, and trying to prevent others from walking into dangers zone, and calling 911 as soon as possible.[32] Everyone should be aware of their environments, as victims are usually random, one should always have an exit plan.

If one cannot get out safely one must find a place to hide, acting quickly and quietly. Turn off lights, lock doors, silence phones, and block doors. If one cannot find safe room, hide behind large objects. Remain quiet and calm and be out of shooters view.

Avoid-Deny-Defend is another plan. This is part of the run, hide, fight plan, which is the fight portion. If one is at risk or alone or as a group, fight and act with aggression, use improvised weapons, and one should commit to their actions, in order to attempt to incapacitate the shooter.

It should also be noted that when help does arrive, first responders are not there to tend to injuries, they are there to incapacitate the shooter, everyone should keep their hands visible, avoid pointing, and know help is coming to the injured.

The Active Shooter Event Quick Reference Guide created by the FBI is something providers should have in their offices and on walls at hospitals[33,34] (**Fig. 4**). There are many other plans as well, a few being the following:

The 4 As Active Shooter Response is a process and acronym to prevent or reduce loss of life.

- Accept that an emergency is happening
- Assess what you can do next so that one can save as many people as possible
- Act by locking and barricading doors, turning off lights, and having people get on the floor and hide or evacuate or fight back. Fighting back is the last resort
- Alert law enforcement and security

ALICE Active Shooter Response is an acronym to increase your chances of surviving a surprise attack.

- Alert via any method possible
- Lockdown if evacuation not possible
- Inform via any means, including social media
- Counter only if being confronted
- Evacuate from danger zone as soon as possible

Window of Life Active Shooter Response is another plan that details similar methods. Providers should take note of these plans and also remind themselves if they are in a situation; they must protect themselves and not rush to provide care if it is not safe. If on the receiving end, at the hospital, providers will need to make difficult calls when many people come into the hospital at one time.[35]

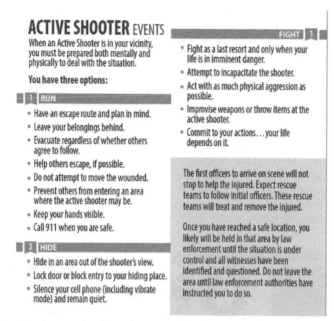

Fig. 4. Active shooter event quick reference guide. Source FBI. (*From* Active Shooter Event Quick Reference Guide — FBI. https://www.fbi.gov/file-repository/active-shooter-event-quick-reference-guide_2015.pdf/view. Accessed May 23, 2019.)

Providers need to also be reminded to change their triage skills; they need to focus on who they can save. The clinician cannot focus on the most critical if they are not able to be saved. At Sunrise Emergency Department (ED) after the Las Vegas shooting, more than 100 people entered the ED on their own in Ubers, taxis, walking in, and relying on random civilians to transport them. Hospitals are starting trainings for preparation for mass casualty incidents.[36] Providers need to assign people to triage in the hospital noting who need the operating room immediately and who can wait. Providers should use the START method, which stands for Simple Triage and Rapid Treatment. Patients are assessed whether or not they are walking, breathing, and how well they are breathing and if they will decline. They are assigned a color, black for deceased, red for critical, yellow for moderate, green for least severe.[37,38]

HEALTH CARE AND GOVERNMENT INITIATIVES

Now is the Time created by President Obama in 2013 on January 16th gave permission to health care providers to submit information to law enforcement if they note a threat. The initiative also gave providers the right to ask if patients have a gun, although as mentioned some states have created laws regarding this. On February 20th, Affordable Care Health Act gave 62 million coverage for mental health services. The Now is the Time campaign implemented background checks for all gun sales and strengthened the background check system. It also limited ammunition magazines to 10 rounds. It also gave money to schools for more police enforcement and funding to research on causes and prevention of gun violence.[39,40]

The Stop the Bleed is a campaign by the Department of Homeland Security. Providers should be familiar with this campaign and educate parents and patients to take this course. The basics are to always remember to make sure your area is safe before rushing to help others. Either you or someone else should be designated to call 911. One should apply steady pressure with the hands or knee in larger areas. Firm, steady pressure should be applied, apply dressings to the area, and continue to hold pressure. If the bleeding is not stopping, one should apply a tourniquet as high on the extremity as possible above the wound. This campaign has been very grass-roots and many schools, places of worship, and commerce are now keeping tourniquets on the walls such as automated external defibrillators.[41] Providers should take a Stop the Bleed Course, teach, or host a course. It is our responsibility to be empowered (**Fig. 5**).

The Office of Justice Programs provides toolkits for victim services, emergency medical services, fire, and law enforcement. The goal here is to make sure to take care of providers who are victims of second-hand trauma. The goal here is to create work environments where providers can speak about what they saw and how the events made them feel. Not all exposure to events is negative. Terms known as vicarious resilience and vicarious transformation are where providers may draw inspiration

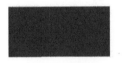
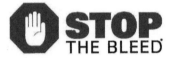

No matter how rapid the arrival of professional emergency responders, bystanders will always be first on the scene. A person who is bleeding can die from blood loss within five minutes, so it's important to quickly stop the blood loss.

Remember to be aware of your surroundings and move yourself and the injured person to safety, if necessary.

Call 911.

Bystanders can take simple steps to keep the injured alive until appropriate medical care is available. Here are three actions that you can take to help save a life:

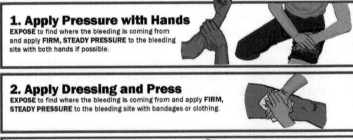

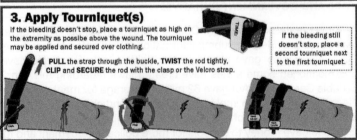

Fig. 5. Stop the bleed: DHS. (*From* Stop the Bleed | Homeland Security. https://www.dhs.gov/stopthebleed. Accessed May 24, 2019.)

from their victim's resilience and it encourages the provider to strengthen their own beliefs. Compassion satisfaction is a term where providers feel a sense of meaning working in the field. The toolkit has more than 500 resources and help recognize if vicarious trauma effects versus resilience are occurring.[42]

The Federal Emergency Management Agency offers in their Emergency Management Institute a course IS-907 on how to respond to an active shooter. This course aids non-law enforcement on how to take charge, recognize workplace violence, understand how to take action to prevent and prepare for active shooters, and learn how to manage consequences of an active shooter incident[43] (https://training.fema.gov/is/courseoverview.aspx?code=IS-907).

Advanced Law Enforcement Rapid Response Training (ALERRT) program created by the FBI trains first responders and medical providers and civilians on active shooters. ALERRT is based out of Texas State and has been awarded more than $72 million in grant money for training.

The FBI's Law Enforcement Enterprise Portal offers a variety of active shooter materials for law enforcement agencies and other first responders to help ensure preparedness for these types of events, including crisis resources, law enforcement training, assistance on dealing with victims, and a directory of FBI field offices to call and report a suspicious person.[44]

A Disaster triage game, 60 seconds to Survival, developed by Dr. Mark Cicero out of Yale University is a video game that teaches providers, students, and laypersons how to triage patients in a mass casualty incident.[45] The game can be found at http://disastertriagegame.org/index.html.

The FBI's Office for Victim Assistance, established in 2001, provides a variety of support services to victims/family members, first responders, investigative teams, and other operational elements. OVA assets available to support active shooter incidents include our field office victim specialists and members of our Victim Assistance Rapid Deployment Team from around the country, who are specially trained to handle mass casualty incidents.

The Congressional Research Service, the FBI, the Mass Shootings in America project by Stanford University all are actively monitoring active shooter events. Methodologies and data collection methods can be found for providers to become more informed on past shooters behaviors.[1]

The Department of Homeland Security (DHS) advises to create a plan for recovery from an active shooter,[46] which includes a short-term and long-term plan. The short-term plan includes the following: account for all personnel and visitors; facilitate medical assistance; contact family members; coordinate with emergency medical services and law enforcement; establish a family assistance area, a way to communicate updated information;, and coordinate people getting their belongings back. The long-term plan includes operations on how to reopen, grief counseling, process worker's compensation or other financial claims, and connecting employees with an assistance program.[46–48]

Virginia Tech student Colin Goddard, who was shot 4 times, created a moving documentary that aired at the Sundance Film Festival: Living for 32. In this film, Colin spoke of his experiences but also detailed with a hidden camera how easy it was to acquire a firearm in America. For years, he served as a senior policy advocate for Everytown for Gun Safety. This organization and Moms Demand Action for Gun Sense are 2 grassroots initiatives where mayors, mothers, teachers, students, survivors, and gun owners have come together with more than 5 million members working toward preventing shootings and lobbying for action against guns violence (https://everytown.org/).

The Department of Homeland Security has also set into action to secure the nation's Soft Targets and Crowded Places (ST-CPs). These include all locations that could be areas of attack. DHS is working with individuals who own stadiums, centers, hospitals, etc. to reduce the number of mass casualties. Individuals interested in working to secure their ST-CP can email NICC@hq.dhs.gov. DHS also has Hometown Security, which empowers the public to connect, plan, train, and report.[49]

The CDC is also keeping data on firearm mortality and tracking of data. The World Health Organization (WHO) has collected data and made recommendations on mass casualty management systems as well as declared violence a public health problem working to educate the public and stop illicit trade of firearms.[50,51] The WHO is also working on preventing and education in the realms on attacks against health care workers. Attacks are occurring at a high rate against health care workers.[52–54] In some countries if health care workers help someone hurt on the government side, rebels are coming in and shooting them (**Fig. 6**).

ARE OTHER COUNTRIES EXPERIENCING THIS?

In November 2015 explosions occurred at the Stade de France just outside of Paris and then within 20 minutes shootings at 4 sites and 3 bloody explosions occurred in the capital. Ten minutes later a massacre takes place and hundreds of people are held hostage at a Paris concert hall. A coordinated White Plan of Action was taken into place. A crisis team of 15 people gathered and they organized triage and mobile teams to the sites composed of a doctor, nurse, and a driver that went to the wounded or to aid other hospitals. The Paris SAMU, the ambulance service, deployed 45 medical teams and 15 in reserve. Off-duty health care employees were mobilized in.[55]

Other countries in Europe and the EU outside of France are experiencing this too. A Cameroon doctor, known for taking care of Ebola was shot dead at a University Hospital in 2019. The massacre in Norway was discusses previously. This is not just a US epidemic (**Table 3**). This is a crisis amongst us all.

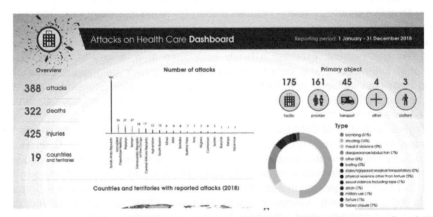

Fig. 6. Shooting attacks on health care workers: 2018. (*From* WHO | Reports and statistics archive. *WHO.* 2019. https://www.who.int/emergencies/attacks-on-health-care/archive/en/. Accessed May 25, 2019.)

Table 3
Mass shootings in Europe and the EU (January 2009–2015)

Year	Month	Day	Location	Country	Fatalities (Not	Nonfatal Injuries
2009	3	11	Winnenden	Germany	13	7
2009	12	31	Espoo	Finland	5	0
2010	6	2	Cumbria	England	12	11
2010	8	30	Devinska Nova Ves	Slovakia	7	15
2011	4	9	Alphen aan den Rijn	Netherlands	6	17
2011	7	22	Oslo and Utoya	Norway	67	110
2011	12	13	Liege	Belgium	6	125
2012	3	19	Toulouse	France	4	0
2012	4	12	Smilkovci	Macedonia	5	0
2012	9	5	Chevaline	France	4	0
2012	11	5	Moscow	Russia	6	1
2013	2	27	Menznau	Switzerland	4	5
2013	4	9	Velika Ivanca	Serbia	13	1
2013	4	22	Belgorod	Russia	6	1
2013	9	16	Annaberg	Austria	4	1
2014	5	24	Brussels	Belgium	4	0
2014	11	3	Tirana	Albania	4	2
2015	1	7	Paris	France	12	11
2015	1	9	Paris	France	4	0
2015	2	24	Uhersky Brod	Czech Republic	9	1
2015	5	10	Wurenlingen	Switzerland	4	0
2015	5	15	Naples	Italy	4	6
2015	5	17	Kanjiza	Serbia	6	0
2015	8	25	Roye	France	4	3
2015	11	13	Paris	France	130	368
				Total Europe	343	685
				EU Total	230	559

From Comparing Death Rates from Mass Public Shootings and Mass Public Violence in the US and Europe. Crime Prevention Research Center, 23 June 2015. https://crimeresearch.org/2015/06/comparing-death-rates-from-mass-public-shootings-in-the-us-and-europe. Accessed May 24, 2019.

SUMMARY

Mass shootings occur on average every 12.5 days in the United States.[23] There is no typical profile for an active shooter. Providers should look out for patients who are depressed and feel bullied. Asking specific questions that focus on the psychiatric review of systems and social history are key elements to helping find out if a patient may be at risk of becoming an active shooter. Providers should also assess the long-term mental health of those affected by mass shootings and ask about RBF and check lead levels. Providers should ask questions related to gun ownership according to their state legislations and document precisely. One should not hesitate to report a suspicious or potentially violent individual whether it be at work or a patient to Law Enforcement or the FBI field offices. HIPPA and FERPA laws protect providers and educators. Providers may be the attacker's first point of contact in a routine medical visit.

Initiatives for training should be sought out; one should have a plan of action if one encounters an active shooter. We all must work together to make our world a safer place (for information on laws see Ref.[56]).

REFERENCES

1. Center for Victims of Crime in partnership with the Office for Victims of Crime N. 2018 NCVRW Resource Guide: Mass Casualty Shootings Fact Sheet. Available at: https://everytownresearch.org/documents/2015/09/analysis-. Accessed May 24, 2019.
2. Gun violence archive. Available at: https://www.gunviolencearchive.org/. Accessed May 23, 2019.
3. Active Shooter Incidents in the United States in 2018 — FBI. Available at: https://www.fbi.gov/file-repository/active-shooter-incidents-in-the-us-2018-041019.pdf/view. Accessed May 23, 2019.
4. Quick Look: 250 Active Shooter Incidents in the United States Between 2000-2017 — FBI. Available at: https://www.fbi.gov/about/partnerships/office-of-partner-engagement/active-shooter-incidents-graphics. Accessed May 23, 2019.
5. Second Amendment | Wex Legal Dictionary/Encyclopedia | LII/Legal Information Institute: Cornell Law School. Available at: https://www.law.cornell.edu/wex/second_amendment. Accessed May 23, 2019.
6. Active Shooter Incidents in the United States in 2016 and 2017 — FBI. Available at: https://www.fbi.gov/file-repository/active-shooter-incidents-us-2016-2017.pdf/view. Accessed May 24, 2019.
7. Making Prevention a Reality: Identifying, Assessing, and Managing the Threat of Targeted Attacks — FBI. Available at: https://www.fbi.gov/file-repository/making-prevention-a-reality.pdf/view. Accessed May 23, 2019.
8. Vossekuil B, Fein R, Reddy M, et al. The final report and findings of the safe school initiative: implications for the prevention of school attacks in the united states united states secret service and United States. Washington, DC: Department of Education; 2004. Available at: https://www2.ed.gov/admins/lead/safety/preventingattacksreport.pdf. Accessed May 23, 2019.
9. COPS Office: Grants and Resources for Community Policing. Available at: https://ric-zai-inc.com/ric.php?page=detail&id=COPS-W0857. Accessed May 23, 2019.
10. A Study of Active Shooter Incidents in the United States Between 2000 and 2013 — FBI. Available at: https://www.fbi.gov/file-repository/active-shooter-study-2000-2013-1.pdf/view. Accessed May 24, 2019.
11. Active Shooter Incidents in the United States in 2014 and 2015 — FBI. Available at: https://www.fbi.gov/file-repository/activeshooterincidentsus_2014-2015.pdf/view. Accessed May 24, 2019.
12. 2000 to 2017 Active Shooter Incidents — FBI. Available at: https://www.fbi.gov/file-repository/active-shooter-incidents-2000-2017.pdf/view. Accessed May 23, 2019.
13. Florida Bill Could Muzzle Doctors On Gun Safety : NPR. Available at: https://www.npr.org/2011/05/07/136063523/florida-bill-could-muzzle-doctors-on-gun-safety. Accessed May 23, 2019.
14. Florida Gov. Rick Scott made it illegal for doctors to talk to patients about guns, TV ad says | PolitiFact Florida. Available at: https://www.politifact.com/florida/statements/2018/feb/22/giffords/florida-gov-rick-scott-made-it-illegal-doctors-tal/. Accessed May 24, 2019.

15. Florida bill: physicians inquiring about firearms. Available at: https://www.myfloridahouse.gov/Sections/Documents/loaddoc.aspx?FileName=h0155z.JDC.DOCX&DocumentType=Analysis&BillNumber=0155&Session=2011. Accessed May 23, 2019.

16. Leiner M, De la Vega I, Johansson B. Deadly mass shootings, mental health, and policies and regulations: what we are obligated to do! Front Pediatr 2018; 6:99.

17. Cabrera JF, Kwon R. Income inequality, household income, and mass shooting in the United States. Front Public Health 2018;6:294.

18. Lin P-I, Fei L, Barzman D, et al. What have we learned from the time trend of mass shootings in the U.S.? PLoS One 2018;13(10):e0204722.

19. Metzl JM, MacLeish KT. Mental illness, mass shootings, and the politics of American firearms. Am J Public Health 2015;105(2):240–9.

20. Was Adam Lanza an Undiagnosed Schizophrenic? | Psychology Today. Available at: https://www.psychologytoday.com/us/blog/we-can-work-it-out/201212/was-adam-lanza-undiagnosed-schizophrenic. Accessed May 23, 2019.

21. Consortium for Risk-Based Firearm Policy. Guns, Public Health, and Mental Illness. Available at: http://efsgv.org/wp-content/uploads/2018/02/Guns-Public-Health-and-Mental-Illness-1.pdf.

22. Philpott-Jones S. Mass shootings, mental illness, and gun control. Hastings Cent Rep 2018;48(2):7–9.

23. Towers S, Gomez-Lievano A, Khan M, et al. Contagion in Mass Killings and School Shootings. PLoS One 2015;10:e0117259.

24. Meindl JN, Ivy JW. Mass shootings: the role of the media in promoting generalized imitation. Am J Public Health 2017;107(3):368–70.

25. Geoffroy PA, Amad A. Seasonal Influence on Mass Shootings. Am J Public Health 2016;106(5):e15–6.

26. Shultz JM, Thoresen S, Galea S. The Las Vegas shootings—underscoring key features of the firearm epidemic. JAMA 2017;318(18):1753.

27. Carli P, Pons F, Levraut J, et al. The French emergency medical services after the Paris and Nice terrorist attacks: what have we learnt? Lancet 2017;390: 2735–8.

28. The Uninjured Victims Of The Virginia Tech Shootings : NPR. Available at: https://www.npr.org/2017/04/14/523042249/the-uninjured-victims-of-the-virginia-tech-shootings. Accessed May 27, 2019.

29. Weiss D, Tomasallo CD, Meiman JG, et al. Elevated blood lead levels associated with retained bullet fragments — United States, 2003–2012. MMWR Morb Mortal Wkly Rep 2017;66(5):130–3.

30. Gun Violence Survivors Face Lead Poisoning From Bullets | Time. Available at: http://time.com/longform/gun-violence-survivors-lead-poisoning/. Accessed June 4, 2019.

31. Sansbury BS, Graves K, Scott W. Managing traumatic stress responses among clinicians: Individual and organizational tools for self-care. Trauma 2015;17(2): 114–22.

32. DHHS, Aspr, Doj, Fema. Incorporating active shooter incident planning into health care facility emergency operations plans. Available at: http://fema.gov. Accessed May 23, 2019.

33. Active Shooter Event Quick Reference Guide — FBI. Available at: https://www.fbi.gov/file-repository/active-shooter-event-quick-reference-guide_2015.pdf/view. Accessed May 23, 2019.

34. How to respond. Available at: https://www.dhs.gov/sites/default/files/publications/active-shooter-pocket-card-508.pdf. Accessed May 23, 2019.

35. Active shooter planning and response in a healthcare setting — FBI. Available at: https://www.fbi.gov/file-repository/active_shooter_planning_and_response_in_a_healthcare_setting.pdf/view. Accessed May 23, 2019.

36. How Hospitals Train to Treat Victims of Mass Shootings | Patient Advice | US News. Available at: https://health.usnews.com/health-care/patient-advice/articles/2018-09-13/how-hospitals-train-to-treat-victims-of-mass-shootings. Accessed May 23, 2019.

37. Benson M, Koenig KL, Schultz CH. Disaster triage: START, then SAVE-a new method of dynamic triage for victims of a catastrophic earthquake. Prehosp Disaster Med 1996;11(2):117–24.

38. Newport Beach CFD. START Support Services. Available at: http://citmt.org/Start/thanks.htm.

39. Now is the time | The White House. Available at: https://obamawhitehouse.archives.gov/issues/preventing-gun-violence. Accessed May 25, 2019.

40. Progress report on the president's executive actions to reduce gun violence. Available at: https://obamawhitehouse.archives.gov/sites/default/files/docs/november_exec_actions_progress_report_final.pdf. Accessed May 25, 2019.

41. Stop the Bleed | Homeland Security. Available at: https://www.dhs.gov/stopthebleed. Accessed May 24, 2019.

42. Vicarious Trauma Toolkit | Tools for Victim Services. Available at: https://vtt.ovc.ojp.gov/tools-for-victim-services. Accessed May 23, 2019.

43. EMI - IS907: Active Shooter: What You Can Do. Available at: https://training.fema.gov/is/courseoverview.aspx?code=IS-907. Accessed May 23, 2019.

44. Law Enforcement Enterprise Portal (LEEP) — FBI. Available at: https://www.fbi.gov/services/cjis/leep. Accessed May 24, 2019.

45. 60 Seconds to Survival. Available at: http://disastertriagegame.org/index.html. Accessed May 24, 2019.

46. First Responder | Homeland Security. Available at: https://www.dhs.gov/cisa/first-responder. Accessed May 23, 2019.

47. Recovering from an Active Shooter Incident; Department of Homeland Security. Available at: https://www.dhs.gov/cisa/active-shooter-preparedness. Accessed May 23, 2019.

48. Active Shooter Preparedness | Homeland Security. Available at: https://www.dhs.gov/cisa/active-shooter-preparedness. Accessed May 24, 2019.

49. Department of Homeland Security U. DHS Soft Target and Crowded Place Security Enhancement and Coordination Plan (20180102). Available at: https://www.dhs.gov/sites/default/files/publications/DHS-Soft-Target-Crowded-Place-Security-Plan-Overview-052018-508_0.pdf. Accessed May 23, 2019.

50. Mass casualty management systems strategies and guidelines for building health sector capacity health action in crises injury and violence prevention. Available at: http://www.who.int/crises. Accessed May 25, 2019.

51. WHO. Small arms and global health. Geneva: WHO; 2014. Available at: https://www.who.int/violence_injury_prevention/publications/violence/small_arms/en/.

52. At Ta Cks on Hea l Th c Are Prevent ● Protect ● Provide. Available at: https://www.who.int/emergencies/attacks-on-health-care/attacks-on-health-care-28November2018.pdf?ua=1. Accessed May 25, 2019.

53. WHO. Violence against health workers. Geneva: WHO; 2018. Available at: https://www.who.int/violence_injury_prevention/violence/workplace/en/. Accessed May 25, 2019.

54. WHO. Reports and statistics archive. Geneva: WHO; 2019. Available at: https://www.who.int/emergencies/attacks-on-health-care/archive/en/. Accessed May 25, 2019.
55. Hirsch M, Carli P, Nizard R, et al. The medical response to multisite terrorist attacks in Paris. Lancet 2015;386:2535–8.
56. Santaella-Tenorio J, Cerdá M, Villaveces A, et al. What do we know about the association between firearm legislation and firearm-related injuries? Epidemiol Rev 2016;38(1):140–57. https://doi.org/10.1093/epirev/mxv012.

Stopping the Bleed:
Hemorrhage Control and Fluid Resuscitation

Andrew D. Fisher, MPAS, PA-C[a,b,*], Brandon M. Carius, MPAS, PA-C[c]

KEYWORDS

- Trauma • Hemorrhage • Tourniquet • Blood transfusion

KEY POINTS

- Hemorrhage is a leading cause of mortality in trauma.
- Limb and junctional hemorrhage are controlled with tourniquets and hemostatic dressings.
- Tranexamic acid is an antifibrinolytic adjunct that may be considered in hemorrhagic shock.
- Whole blood and balanced component blood transfusions have demonstrated benefit over crystalloid and high red blood cell transfusions.
- The use of resuscitative endovascular balloon occlusion of the aorta (REBOA) may be an option for critically injured patients in a disaster or mass casualty.

INTRODUCTION

Traumatic hemorrhage accounts for up to 20% of potentially survivable (PS) deaths in the United States.[1] Many of these deaths could be prevented if proper care is applied immediately. A stepwise progression, from layperson hemorrhage control to advanced resuscitative care in the hospital, are all critical to decrease PS deaths. Since 9/11, several significant changes were made to the approach to trauma care. Many of these changes are based on advancements in prehospital care refined in the conflicts in Iraq, Syria, and Afghanistan. The approach is based on anatomic regions, primarily separated into the limbs, junctional areas, and noncompressible torso hemorrhage (NCTH). In this article we discuss how to assess and treat life-threatening hemorrhage in each of these areas.

Disclaimer: Opinions or assertions contained herein are the private views of the authors and are not to be construed as official or as reflecting the views of the Texas A&M College of Medicine, the Department of the Army, the Defense Health Agency, or the Department of Defense.
Disclosures: The authors declare no conflicts of interest.
a Medical Command, Texas Army National Guard, Austin, TX, USA; b Texas A&M College of Medicine, Temple, TX, USA; c San Antonio Military Medical Center, 3551 Roger Brooke Drive, JBSA Fort Sam Houston, TX 78234
* Corresponding author. 2401 S. 31st Street Temple, TX 76508.
E-mail address: andrewdfisher@icloud.com

LIMB HEMORRHAGE

Of all PS injuries, limb hemorrhage is most significantly decreased with bleeding control training. Combat experiences in Iraq and Afghanistan produced multiple studies demonstrating the benefit of tourniquets to control limb hemorrhage.[2–5] However, these were hard lessons learned. It has been known for many years that massive hemorrhage from a limb is a PS death. Dr J.S. Maughon, a Navy surgeon during the Vietnam War, remarked in 1970 that "little if any improvement has been made in treatment of combat wounds in the past 100 years."[6] Even more astonishing, no significant changes were made for 31 years following this declaration. As the wars in Afghanistan and Iraq began in 2001 and 2003, combat medics still relied on Civil War vintage pain management relying largely on morphine and recommended tourniquets only as a last resort for hemorrhage control.[7] This antiquated thinking occurred despite development of the Tactical Combat Casualty Care (TCCC) curriculum, which focused on decreasing prehospital combat deaths through an emphasis on early hemorrhage control that included tourniquets.

After the conflict in Mogadishu in 1993 (captured in the movie Blackhawk Down), the 75th Ranger Regiment and other US special operations forces units were identified areas of opportunity to train for combat casualties after an extensive medical after action review.[8] About the same time, Butler and colleagues[9] published their article "Tactical Combat Casualty Care in Special Operations," which outlined identifying and treating combat wounded. Only a few units implemented TCCC before 9/11 with a focus on proficient tactical medicine. Butler and colleagues placed heavy emphasis on identifying and treating major causes of preventable death, especially early tourniquet application for effective bleeding control.

Of the units to implement TCCC before 9/11, the 75th Ranger Regiment was able to make TCCC and medical training part of the unit's culture. Because of this, they were able to subsequently eliminate PS deaths in the prehospital setting, a feat never before accomplished in the history of combat.[2] Elsewhere in special operations, the PS mortality rate was 15% (N = 82), with three dying from limb hemorrhage,[10] whereas the rest of the Department of Defense maintained about a 25% PS mortality rate.[11] The 75th Ranger Regiment followed the recommendations from TCCC for hemorrahge, using either the Combat Application Tourniquet® ([C-A-T] North American Rescue, Greer, SC) and the SOF® Tactical Tourniquet ([SOF®TT], Anderson, SC). After the mass implementation of tourniquets for massive hemorrhage throughout the force, there was a 67% decrease in death due to limb hemorrhage.[7] Currently, there are a total of 10 tourniquets recommended for use in TCCC and the prehospital setting.

The lessons learned through the use of limb tourniquets for bleeding control rapidly spread from these combat foundations into civilian medical practice. For many years, similar to the military, the use of tourniquets for hemorrhage control was perceived to be a last resort of treatment. This was based on poor science and anecdotal evidence. However, in part because of the extended length of current conflicts, there were military physicians, such as retired Colonel John B. Holcomb, who effectively transitioned to civilian practice, bringing experiences and techniques with them.[12] This helped bring the concept of aggressive hemorrhage control with limb tourniquets back to the forefront. By 2007, civilian use of limb tourniquets was being discussed and implemented.[13–16] In turn, the early use of tourniquets, either prehospital or in the emergency room, has demonstrated a decrease in blood product use and a survival benefit when compared with tourniquets placed at the trauma center (odds ratio, 4.5; 95% confidence interval, 1.23–16.4; $P = .02$).[17]

Effective prehospital care became more visible when, on December 14, 2012, the United States witnessed a gunman kill 20 children and 6 adults at the Sandy Hook Elementary School in Newtown, Connecticut. Although none of the deaths could have been prevented with tourniquet application, this tragedy nevertheless sparked a significant civilian initiative. In April 2013, The Hartford Consensus was published from a committee made up of diverse stakeholders including the American College of Surgeons (ACS), Department of Defense, Department of Homeland Security, Health and Human Services Assistant Secretary for Preparedness and Response, and the American College of Emergency Physicians.[18] The resulting protocol provided instruction for bystanders should someone find themselves in a situation requiring bleeding control, to include mass shooting situations. This instruction laid the foundations for the establishment of the Stop the Bleed (STB) campaign and the Bleeding Control Basics (B-Con) course.[19] These efforts sought to empower bystanders to control traumatic hemorrhage before the arrival of emergency medical services. Furthermore, the development of bleedingcontrol.org allowed for a central online repository of information for instructors and students. The STB campaign began as a grassroots movement, with little funding to support courses and instructor credentialing. In 2017, a call to action was announced by military medics and veterans, announcing the first National Stop the Bleed Day that would take place on March 31, 2018. They used social media to fuel the movement and sought support from the ACS, the federal government, and other stakeholders. The movement became incredibly successful, training more than 43,000 people in hemorrhage control techniques over a 2-week period from March 26 to April 7, 2018.[20] The success of these efforts promoted the group to move the dates of National Stop the Bleed Day to the entire month of May and rebrand it as National Stop the Bleed Month (http://stopthebleedmonth.org/).

JUNCTIONAL HEMORRHAGE AND HEMOSTATIC DRESSINGS

As a solution for death caused by limb hemorrhage began to spread throughout the military and spilling into the civilian sector, junctional hemorrhage concerns became another target to reduce PS deaths. Junctional hemorrhage is defined as compressible hemorrhage occurring at the junction of an extremity with the torso, where a limb tourniquet is not effective; it also includes the base of the neck.[21] Junctional hemorrhage is treatable by laypersons, although the skills are more difficult to master than the use of a limb tourniquet in massive hemorrhage. Because junctional wounds are not amenable to a limb tourniquet, effective wound packing is critical. The recommended packing materials for junctional hemorrhage are hemostatic dressings.

Early models of hemostatic dressings have significantly evolved into current products. The HemCon bandage (HemCon Medical Technologies, Portland, OR) was first released in 2003 and was the mainstay until QuickClot granules (Z-Medica, Wallingford, CT) were added to the TCCC recommended list in 2006.[22] The HemCon Bandage came as a single sided 4" × 4" or 2" × 2" wafer, which effectively cross-linked red blood cells (RBC) to form a mucoadhesive barrier. QuickClot granules made from volcanic rock (zeolite) came packaged as a powder to be poured into the wound, which would rapidly absorb water to better concentrate clotting factors. However, HemCon and QuickClot granules were initially met with harsh criticism. Because HemCon was a wafer, it could not be packed into a wound like gauze. QuickClot granules produced an exothermic reaction, which was found to burn patients.[22]

In 2008, as technology improved, Z-Medica was able to impregnate gauze with kaolin, a clay mineral that activates the intrinsic coagulation pathway, and market QuikClot Combat Gauze as a replacement for the first-generation hemostatic dressings.[23] Not far behind, CELOX gauze (SAM Medical, Tualatin, OR), HemCon gauze, and ChitoFlex gauze (HemCon Medical Technologies) came onto the market, all being chitosan-based products. Newer versions of these products have largely maintained their original mechanisms.

Hemostatic dressing efficacy has been historically promising in animal studies.[23–26] The use in humans has been demonstrated as safe.[22] Although not demonstrating a significant survival benefit in analysis of the Department of Defense Trauma Registry, outcome data may be confounded because hemostatic dressings are used in more severely wounded patients.[27,28] The Israeli Defense Force prospectively evaluated the use of QuikClot Combat Gauze in 122 patients. Hemostasis was achieved in 88.6% of the junctional hemorrhage and in 91.9% of the extremity hemorrhage.[29] Chitosan-based products have demonstrated effective hemorrhage control in patients on anticoagulants.[30] From these data, hemostatic dressings demonstrate likely benefit for wounds not amenable to limb tourniquets or those that can be packed for limb tourniquet conversion.

Junctional hemorrhage, although not as prevalent as limb hemorrhage in the prehospital setting, is nevertheless a significant contributor to death. The approach junctional hemorrhage should be generally the same, with aggressive use of hemostatic dressings and junctional tourniquets if available. These basic skills and treatments could benefit a great number of patients in a disaster or mass casualty event.

NONCOMPRESSIBLE TORSO HEMORRHAGE

NCTH is the leading cause of PS death.[11,31] The definition of NCTH as described by Morrison and Rasmussen[32] is the vascular disruption in one or more of the following: named axial torso vessel, solid organ injury with grade 4 or greater with shock (systolic blood pressure <90 mm Hg) or immediate operation, thoracic cavity, or pelvic fracture with ring disruption. These injuries are inherently more lethal because pressure cannot be applied to the wound for effective hemorrhage control. In the prehospital setting, effective treatment of NCTH includes tranexamic acid (TXA); blood components, specifically whole blood (WB); and resuscitative balloon occlusion of the aorta (REBOA). Unfortunately, these injuries are almost entirely untreatable by bystanders and first responders, and effective treatment therefore relies less on provision of first aid than on rapid transport to definitive medical care.

TRANEXAMIC ACID

TXA is a lysine analogue that prevents plasminogen conversion to plasmin, in turn delaying the onset of physiologic fibrinolysis (blood clot breakdown). Although the Food and Drug Administration initially approved TXA for hemophilia-associated bleeding with dental procedures in 1986 and later for heavy menstrual bleeding in 2009,[33] the use of TXA in trauma patients anticipated to require blood transfusion remains an off-label use in the United States.[34] It continues to be used for trauma patients throughout the globe, most prominently in Europe. TXA came to prominence in 2010 after the Clinical Randomization of an Antifibrinolytic in Significant Hemorrhage 2 (CRASH-2) study. This large multinational investigation involving more than 20,000 patients evaluated the impact of TXA on mortality, vascular occlusive events, and blood transfusion because of trauma.[34] The results demonstrated an overall mortality benefit, with rates of 14.5% versus 16.0% in the TXA and control group, respectively, with a relative risk of 0.91 (95% confidence interval, 0.85–0.97; $P = .0035$).

The Military Application of Tranexamic Acid in Trauma Emergency Resuscitation (MATTERs) trial established the first substantial evaluation of TXA in the combat setting. From 896 evaluated patients, investigators examined mortality benefits of TXA in a severely traumatized population. The use of TXA demonstrated lower unadjusted mortality (17.4% vs 23.9%; P = .03), benefiting those receiving a massive transfusion the most (14.4% vs 28.1%; P = .004).[35] In a second evaluation of the same data, investigators published MATTERs II, demonstrating a survival benefit when using cryoprecipitate with TXA (n = 258) with 11.6% mortality compared with those who did not receive TXA (23.6%).[36] However, similar combat-focused studies failed to identify a survival benefit of TXA administration, although this set of conclusions were likely limited by smaller populations.[37] A recent meta-analysis of more than 40,000 patients demonstrated a 10% decrease in mortality benefit for every 15-minute delay in TXA administration.[38] This finding is critical to ensure quick administration of TXA in a hemorrhaging patient. Current recommendations state an initial dosage of 1 gram of TXA infused over 10 minutes, with a second dose infused over 8 hours. Additional dosage and administration recommendations are currently being investigated.

BLOOD PRODUCTS

The use of whole blood (WB) for trauma resuscitation has been around for 100 years. In the early 1900s, Carl Landsteiner discovered the ABO system, which matched blood groups for transfusion, effectively making the process safer.[39] Leading up to the World War I, the use of a basic preservative solution allowed WB to be stored until it was needed.[40,41] This ability helped establish the foundations of modern day blood banking. Likewise, successful WB-based resuscitation in World War I firmly established its initial role in the treatment of traumatic hemorrhage.[42]

As the world plunged into World War II, the continued use of WB transfusions for trauma further established its safety and efficacy. In 1941, the Rhesus (Rh) antigen was discovered and would further help effectively match blood types to make WB transfusions safer.[43] Despite the recognition of ABO and Rh, most blood transfusions were group O.[44] There was ongoing evaluation of titers in group O WB. Researchers noted that when the levels of IgM anti-A and anti-B were lower than 1:512, there were fewer reactions.

In 1944, a patient was transfused 75 mL of group O WB with an IgM anti-A titer of 1:8000. The reaction was severe, but the casualty survived. This event along with previous studies demonstrating fewer reactions with titer levels below 1:512, the Army Blood Program declared low titer group O WB (LTOWB) as IgM anti-A and anti-B less than 1:256.[44] The practice of LTOWB was carried forward to the Korean War, where more than 400,000 units of LTOWB was transfused without significant transfusion reactions.[45]

The use of whole blood (FWB) is now making a comeback for trauma resuscitation. In the early years of the wars in Iraq and Afghanistan, combat support hospitals began using fresh whole blood as they depleted the supplies of blood components. The use of FWB demonstrated decreased mortality and better outcomes when compared to component therapy.[46] Currently, over 10,000 units of FWB have been transfused.[47] In 2015, the Committee on Tactical Combat Casualty Care (CoTCCC) recommended the use of WB in the prehospital setting.[48]

As the CoTCCC made the recommendation for the use of WB in the prehospital combat setting, units within the military began to develop and implement a LTOWB, with the intent of using it as FWB. As the program matured, units of LTOWB collected in the US were shipped to units in Afghanistan.[49] The US military used titer levels previously utilized, IgM anti – A and anti – B titer <256. While the US military has their defined titer levels, the civilian community can differ. It varies from IgM anti – A and anti – B titer between 1:50 and 1:256.[50] There is no international definition of low titer group O whole blood.

The use of LTOWB is now in many hospital and prehospital programs. The Southwest Texas Regional Advisory Council (STRAC) has implemented LTOWB for an area 26,000 square miles in southwest Texas.[51] These efforts are promising, as the use of LTOWB in hemorrhagic shock offers—one product, doesn't make things worse, and gives what the patient is losing.

The prevalence of low titer donors also vary, from an Armed Serviced Blood Program study, a total of 2237 participating soldiers, 69.5% of donors met low titer donor criteria on the first test, but in those tested more than once, there was a tendency to become low titer over time.[52] In south Texas, of male O D+ donors, 2848 (86.99%) tested as low titer for IgM anti – A or –B.[53] LTOWB has limitations, after about 14 days, there is decreased PLT function.[54] This may be mitigated by using cold stored platelets with WB.

Despite the demonstrated safety and benefit of WB, after the Vietnam War there was a shift to the use of crystalloids for trauma resuscitation, especially in the prehospital setting. Earlier versions of advanced trauma life support (ATLS) recommended that patients be administered 2 L of crystalloids before transfusing RBCs.[55] Several studies have since demonstrated superior outcomes with less crystalloid and using WB or a balanced ratio of RBCs, plasma, and platelets in 1:1:1 to replicate WB.[56–59] More recently, the ATLS guidelines have reflected this evidence and called for a more balanced approach, but still recommend 1 L of crystalloid for an initial attempt at intravenous fluid resuscitation. ATLS guidelines still recommends crystalloids in the prehospital setting.

If WB is not immediately available the use of component therapy is preferred over crystalloids. Shackelford and colleagues[60] demonstrated a six-fold early survival benefit when any blood component is given within 34 minutes of injury. Prehospital RBC transfusion has been associated with increased survival at 24 hours, lower odds of shock, and lower transfusion requirements.[61,62] A recent push toward a plasma-first resuscitation approach has produced mixed results thus far. Moore and colleagues[63] failed to demonstrate any benefit when plasma was used on ground ambulances. The study was helpful in the continuing research of prehospital trauma resuscitation. However, the study was criticized for not using prethawed plasma and focusing on long-term mortality outcomes.[64] The Prehospital Air Medical Plasma (PAMPer) study compared plasma with standard treatment, which included crystalloid and RBCs, and demonstrated a 39% risk reduction in mortality with plasma first-resuscitation.[65]

Temperature-controlled blood products may have limited use in disasters. Lyophilized (freeze dried) plasma and fresh WB may therefore offer solutions for mass casualty events and disaster medicine. Freeze dried plasma was used in World War II and is credited for saving numerous lives as a prehospital resuscitative fluid.[66] The French have used a modern version since 1994, and it has also been used by the US military and Israeli Defense Force in combat theaters with success.[67–69]

Other treatment modalities, such as recombinant factor VIIa and albumin, have caused more detriment than once thought in trauma resuscitation. The use of recombinant factor VIIa in combat led to increased pulmonary embolisms. The use of fibrinogen, cryoprecipitate, and early administration of calcium may offer benefits for patients requiring a massive transfusion.

RESUSCITATIVE BALLOON OCCLUSION OF THE AORTA

Concerted focus has recently been dedicated to the examination of those patients manifesting junctional hemorrhage and/or NCTH with PS death if more rapidly delivered to definitive operative care. To help transition these patients to the operating table, the concept of REBOA is being implemented and refined for prehospital care. REBOA consists of placing a 7-French catheter sheath into the common femoral artery, then passing a long catheter through to the thoracic aorta and inflating a balloon to stop blood flow below the balloon. This technique essentially establishes an internal cross-clamp effect. REBOA was first described by Carl Hughes in 1954 in Korea where he performed the procedure on three casualties.[70] Although the casualties eventually died from their injuries, Hughes demonstrated the effectiveness of REBOA for temporizing life in transport to operative care.

The pre-endovascular era was not favorable for REBOA use. Two studies from the 1980s demonstrated poor outcomes. Low and colleagues[71] had 13% survival in 15 trauma patients after REBOA and Gupta and colleagues[72] had 35% survival in 20 trauma patients after REBOA. As technology and training improved, however, endovascular capabilities were formally established to increase capabilities.[73]

Research from animal studies helped established REBOA feasibility. White and colleagues[74] found REBOA increases central perfusion pressures with less physiologic disturbance than thoracotomy with aortic clamping in a model of hemorrhagic shock. Morrison and colleagues[75] found in a swine study that overall mortality for complete REBOA was 25%, intermittent REBOA was 37.5%, and no REBOA groups was 100%. They concluded REBOA can temporize exsanguinating hemorrhage and restore life-sustaining perfusion to vital organs, bridging patient care en route to definitive hemorrhage control. Another Morrison study, a retrospective analysis, found that 20% of the 165 UK casualties could have benefited from REBOA, with 89 benefiting from early (prehospital) REBOA.[76]

REBOA was more formally described as a procedure by Stannard and colleagues.[77] They described the technique from access to removal in five steps: (1) arterial access, (2) balloon selection and positioning, (3) balloon inflation, (4) balloon deflation, and (5) sheath removal.[77] They also discussed where the balloon should be placed and described these areas as zones.[77] Zone 1 begins just above the celiac artery and extends to the of the left subclavian artery. Zone II is considered an area of no-occlusion and extends from the celiac artery to the ronal arteries. Finally, zone III extends from the lowest renal artery to the aortic bifurcation.

From the Aortic Occlusion in Resuscitation for Trauma and Acute Care Surgery Registry (AORTA) trial, emerging data suggest that REBOA outcomes are optimal when used in hypotensive patients with noncompressible hemorrhage before loss of signs of life, most likely in the prehospital setting.[78] DuBose and colleagues[78] astutely that if providers are waiting until patients required CPR, no matter your intervention, patients die. Newer animal studies demonstrate increased potential for partial REBOA and/or intermittent REBOA.[79] This approach to REBOA may make it feasible to use in austere and far forward environments.

Movement of REBOA to outside the hospital began with the London Air Ambulance. The first published case of prehospital REBOA was a zone III placement for a pelvic fracture.[80] Since then, the Service d'Aide Medicale Urgente in France and prehospital agencies in Japan have begun to implement and use REBOA.[81–83]

Perhaps the greatest benefit of prehospital REBOA would be in combat. The Air Force special operation surgical team is showing that even physicians without any training can perform REBOA.[84] It is important to highlight that these providers are not vascular, trauma, or acute care surgeons, but general surgeons and noncritical care trained emergency medicine providers. Despite these outcomes, the ACS and American College of Emergency Physicians published a joint statement that states that only critical care trained people should be using REBOA.[85,86] Other international militaries have also developed REBOA for prehospital and austere environments.[87,88] In the United States, although REBOA has been used by many inside the hospital for several years, the prehospital programs are just now starting to be implemented. Although there have been successes, caution is warranted given currently small datasets.

SUMMARY

Although substantial material innovation improves hemorrhage control in the prehospital setting, including that of disasters, it continues to be a significant problem despite decreases in PS death. Fundamentals of hemorrhage control necessitate effective tourniquet placement on bleeding limbs and effective packing and pressure on extremity and nonextremity wounds. The use of TXA to prevent clot breakdown adds intravascular benefit to topical hemostatic agents working extravascularly. Fluid resuscitation using WB or component therapy in a 1:1:1 ratio has shown success in combat theaters and civilian trauma centers, and similar benefit in the civilian prehospital environment. Although new to the prehospital setting, REBOA is possible for implementation and demonstrates mortality benefit with substantial promise if properly incorporated into protocols. However, to be effective, any prehospital intervention must have clearly defined protocols as part of ongoing damage control resuscitation to ensure best outcomes in trauma patients.

REFERENCES

1. National Academies of Sciences E, Medicine. A national trauma care system: integrating military and civilian trauma systems to achieve zero preventable deaths after injury. Washington, DC: The National Academies Press; 2016.
2. Kotwal RS, Montgomery HR, Kotwal BM, et al. Eliminating preventable death on the battlefield. Arch Surg 2011;146(12):1350–8.
3. Kragh JF Jr, Littrel ML, Jones JA, et al. Battle casualty survival with emergency tourniquet use to stop limb bleeding. J Emerg Med 2011;41(6):590–7.
4. Kragh JF Jr, Walters TJ, Baer DG, et al. Survival with emergency tourniquet use to stop bleeding in major limb trauma. Ann Surg 2009;249(1):1–7.
5. Pannell D, Brisebois R, Talbot M, et al. Causes of death in Canadian Forces members deployed to Afghanistan and implications on tactical combat casualty care provision. J Trauma 2011;71(5 Suppl 1):S401–7.
6. Maughon JS. An inquiry into the nature of wounds resulting in killed in action in Vietnam. Mil Med 1970;135(1):8–13.
7. Butler FK. Two decades of saving lives on the battlefield: tactical combat casualty care turns 20. Mil Med 2017;182(3):e1563–8.
8. Mabry RL, Holcomb JB, Baker AM, et al. United States Army Rangers in Somalia: an analysis of combat casualties on an urban battlefield. J Trauma 2000;49(3):515–29.
9. Butler FK, Haymann J, Butler EG. Tactical combat casualty care in special operations. Mil Med 1996;161(Suppl 3):3–16.
10. Holcomb JB, McMullin NR, Pearse L, et al. Causes of death in U.S. Special Operations Forces in the global war on terrorism: 2001-2004. Ann Surg 2007;245(6):986–91.
11. Eastridge BJ, Mabry RL, Seguin P, et al. Death on the battlefield (2001-2011): implications for the future of combat casualty care. J Trauma 2012;73(6, Supplement 5):S431–7.

12. Holcomb JB. 2019. Available at: https://www.utphysicians.com/provider/john-b-holcomb/. Accessed June 19, 2019.

13. Lee C, Porter KM, Hodgetts TJ. Tourniquet use in the civilian prehospital setting. Emerg Med J 2007;24(8):584–7.

14. Doyle GS, Taillac PP. Tourniquets: a review of current use with proposals for expanded prehospital use. Prehosp Emerg Care 2008;12(2):241–56.

15. Dorlac WC, DeBakey ME, Holcomb JB, et al. Mortality from isolated civilian penetrating extremity injury. J Trauma 2005;59(1):217–22.

16. Scerbo MH, Mumm JP, Gates K, et al. Safety and appropriateness of tourniquets in 105 civilians. Prehosp Emerg Care 2016;20(6):712–22.

17. Scerbo MH, Holcomb JB, Taub E, et al. The trauma center is too late: major limb trauma without a pre-hospital tourniquet has increased death from hemorrhagic shock. J Trauma Acute Care Surg 2017;83(6):1165–72.

18. Jacobs LM, McSwain NE Jr, Rotondo MF, et al. Improving survival from active shooter events: the Hartford Consensus. J Trauma Acute Care Surg 2013; 74(6):1399–400.

19. Rasmussen TE, Baer DG, Goolsby C. The giving back: battlefield lesson to national preparedness. J Trauma Acute Care Surg 2016;80(1):166–7.

20. Fisher AD, Carius BM, Lacroix J, et al. National Stop the Bleed Day: the impact of a social media campaign on the Stop the Bleed program. J Trauma Acute Care Surg 2019;87(1):S40–3.

21. Kotwal RS, Butler FK, Gross KR, et al. Management of junctional hemorrhage in tactical combat casualty care: TCCC guidelines? Proposed change 13-03. J Spec Oper Med 2013;13(4):85–93.

22. Bennett BL, Littlejohn LF, Kheirabadi BS, et al. Management of external hemorrhage in TCCC: chitosan-based hemostatic gauze dressings TCCC guidelines - change 13-05. J Spec Oper Med 2014;14(3):12–29.

23. Littlejohn L, Bennett BL, Drew B. Application of current hemorrhage control techniques for backcountry care: part two, hemostatic dressings and other adjuncts. Wilderness Environ Med 2015;26(2):246–54.

24. Johnson D, Bates S, Nukalo S, et al. The effects of QuikClot Combat Gauze on hemorrhage control in the presence of hemodilution and hypothermia. Ann Med Surg (Lond) 2014;3(2):21–5.

25. Kheirabadi BS, Scherer MR, Estep JS, et al. Determination of efficacy of new hemostatic dressings in a model of extremity arterial hemorrhage in swine. J Trauma 2009;67(3):450–9 [discussion: 459–60].

26. Arnaud F, Parreno-Sadalan D, Tomori T, et al. Comparison of 10 hemostatic dressings in a groin transection model in swine. J Trauma 2009;67(4):848–55.

27. Schauer SG, April MD, Naylor JF, et al. Prehospital application of hemostatic agents in Iraq and Afghanistan. Prehosp Emerg Care 2018;22(5):614–23.

28. Schauer SG, April MD, Naylor JF, et al. QuikClot combat gauze use by ground forces in Afghanistan. J Spec Oper Med 2017;17(2):100–5.

29. Shina A, Lipsky AM, Nadler R, et al. Prehospital use of hemostatic dressings by the Israel Defense Forces medical corps: a case series of 122 patients. J Trauma Acute Care Surg 2015;79(4 Suppl 2):S204–9.

30. Chiara O, Cimbanassi S, Bellanova G, et al. A systematic review on the use of topical hemostats in trauma and emergency surgery. BMC Surg 2018;18(1):68.

31. Kisat M, Morrison JJ, Hashmi ZG, et al. Epidemiology and outcomes of noncompressible torso hemorrhage. J Surg Res 2013;184(1):414–21.

32. Morrison JJ, Rasmussen TE. Noncompressible torso hemorrhage: a review with contemporary definitions and management strategies. Surg Clin North Am 2012;92(4):843–58, vii.

33. Napolitano LM, Cohen MJ, Cotton BA, et al. Tranexamic acid in trauma: how should we use it? J Trauma Acute Care Surg 2013;74(6):1575–86.

34. Shakur H, Roberts I, Bautista R, et al. Effects of tranexamic acid on death, vascular occlusive events, and blood transfusion in trauma patients with significant haemorrhage (CRASH-2): a randomised, placebo-controlled trial. Lancet 2010;376:23–32.

35. Morrison JJ, Dubose JJ, Rasmussen TE, et al. Military application of tranexamic acid in trauma emergency resuscitation (MATTERs) study. Arch Surg 2012; 147(2):113–9.

36. Morrison JJ, Ross JD, Dubose JJ, et al. Association of cryoprecipitate and tranexamic acid with improved survival following wartime injury: findings from the MATTERs II Study. JAMA Surg 2013;148(3):218–25.

37. Howard JT, Stockinger ZT, Cap AP, et al. Military use of tranexamic acid in combat trauma. J Trauma Acute Care Surg 2017;83(4):579–88.

38. Gayet-Ageron A, Prieto-Merino D, Ker K, et al. Effect of treatment delay on the effectiveness and safety of antifibrinolytics in acute severe haemorrhage: a meta-analysis of individual patient-level data from 40 138 bleeding patients. Lancet 2018;391(10116):125–32.

39. Schwarz HP, Dorner F. Karl Landsteiner and his major contributions to haematology. Br J Haematol 2003;121:556–65.

40. Robertson OH. Transfusion with preserved red blood cells. Br Med J 1918; 1(2999):691–5.

41. Mollison PL. The introduction of citrate as an anticoagulant for transfusion and of glucose as a red cell preservative. Br J Haematol 2000;108:13–8.

42. Robertson B. Further observations on the results of blood transfusion in war surgery. Ann Surg 1918;67(1):1–13.

43. Kendrick DB. Blood program in World War II. Washington, DC: Office of the Surgeon General; 1964.

44. Berseus O, Boman K, Nessen SC, et al. Risks of hemolysis due to anti-A and anti-B caused by the transfusion of blood or blood components containing ABO-incompatible plasma. Transfusion 2013;53(Suppl 1):114S–23S.

45. Spinella PC, Pidcoke HF, Strandenes G, et al. Whole blood for hemostatic resuscitation of major bleeding. Transfusion 2016;56(Suppl 2):S190–202.

46. Spinella PC, Perkins JG, Grathwohl KW, et al. Warm fresh whole blood is independently associated with improved survival for patients with combat-related traumatic injuries. J Trauma 2009;66(4 Suppl):S69–76.

47. Cap AP, Beckett A, Benov A, et al. Whole blood transfusion. Mil Med 2018; 183(suppl_2):44–51.

48. Butler FK, Holcomb JB, Schreiber MA, et al. Fluid resuscitation for hemorrhagic shock in tactical combat casualty care: TCCC guidelines change 14-01– 2 June 2014. J Spec Oper Med 2014;14(3):30–55.

49. Warner N, Zheng J, Nix G, et al. Prehospital use of group O low titre whole blood. J Spec Oper Med 2018;18(1):15–8.

50. Yazer MH, Spinella PC. Review of low titre group O whole blood use for massively bleeding patients around the world in 2019. ISBT Science Series 2019.

51. McGinity AC, Zhu CS, Greebon L, et al. Pre-hospital low titer cold stored whole blood: philosophy for ubiquitous utilization of O positive product for emergency

use in hemorrhage due to injury. J Trauma Acute Care Surg 2018;6S(Suppl 1): S115–9.

52. Bailey JD, Fisher AD, Yazer MH, et al. Changes in donor antibody titer levels over time in a military group O low-titer whole blood program. Transfusion 2019;59(S2): 1499–506.

53. Beddard R, Ngamsuntikul S, Wafford T, et al. Immunoglobulin M anti-A and anti-B titers in South Texas group O D+ male donors. Transfusion 2019;59(7):2207–10.

54. Dodge M, et al. Whole blood in EMS may save lives. J Emerg Med Serv 2018;50–5.

55. Advanced trauma life support (ATLS(R)): the ninth edition. J Trauma Acute Care Surg 2013;74(5):1363–6.

56. Holcomb JB, Tilley BC, Baraniuk S, et al. Transfusion of plasma, platelets, and red blood cells in a 1:1:1 vs a 1:1:2 ratio and mortality in patients with severe trauma: the PROPPR randomized clinical trial. JAMA 2015;313(5):471–82.

57. Holcomb JB, Jenkins D, Rhee P, et al. Damage control resuscitation: directly addressing the early coagulopathy of trauma. J Trauma 2007;62(2):307–10.

58. Spinella PC, Perkins JG, Grathwohl KW, et al. Warm fresh whole blood is independently associated with improved survival for patients with combat-related traumatic injuries. J Trauma 2009;66(4 Suppl):S69–76.

59. Haut ER, Kalish BT, Cotton BA, et al. Prehospital intravenous fluid administration is associated with higher mortality in trauma patients: a National Trauma Data Bank analysis. Ann Surg 2011;253(2):371–7.

60. Shackelford SA, Del Junco DJ, Powell-Dunford N, et al. Association of prehospital blood product transfusion during medical evacuation of combat casualties in Afghanistan with acute and 30-day survival. JAMA 2017;318(16):1581–91.

61. Brown JB, Cohen MJ, Minei JP, et al. Pretrauma center red blood cell transfusion is associated with reduced mortality and coagulopathy in severely injured patients with blunt trauma. Ann Surg 2015;261(5):997–1005.

62. Brown JB, Sperry JL, Fombona A, et al. Pre-trauma center red blood cell transfusion is associated with improved early outcomes in air medical trauma patients. J Am Coll Surg 2015;220(5):797–808.

63. Moore HB, Moore EE, Chapman MP, et al. Plasma-first resuscitation to treat haemorrhagic shock during emergency ground transportation in an urban area: a randomised trial. The Lancet 2018;392(10144):283–91.

64. Naumann DN, Doughty H, Cotton BA. No gains with plasma-first resuscitation in urban settings? Lancet 2018;392(10144):255–6.

65. Sperry JL, Guyette FX, Brown JB, et al. Prehospital plasma during air medical transport in trauma patients at risk for hemorrhagic shock. N Engl J Med 2018; 379(4):315–26.

66. Beecher HK. Pain in men wounded in battle. Ann Surg 1946;123(2):96–105.

67. Glassberg E, Nadler R, Rasmussen TE, et al. Point-of-injury use of reconstituted freeze dried plasma as a resuscitative fluid: a special report for prehospital trauma care. J Trauma Acute Care Surg 2013;75(2 Suppl 2):S111–4.

68. Martinaud C, Ausset S, Deshayes AV, et al. Use of freeze-dried plasma in French intensive care unit in Afghanistan. J Trauma 2011;71(6):1761–4 [discussion: 1764–5].

69. Cap AP, Pidcoke HF, Spinella P, et al. Damage control resuscitation. Mil Med 2018;183(suppl_2):36–43.

70. Hughes CW. Use of an intra-aortic balloon catheter tamponade for controlling intraabdominal hemorrhage in man. Surgery 1954;36:65–8.

71. Low RB, Longmore W, Rubinstein R, et al. Preliminary report on the use of the Percluder occluding aortic balloon in human beings. Ann Emerg Med 1986;5(12): 1466–9.

72. Gupta BK, Khaneja SC, Flores L, et al. The role of intra-aortic balloon occlusion in penetrating abdominal trauma. J Trauma 1989;29(6):861–5.

73. Fisher AD, Teeter WA, Cordova C, et al. The role i resuscitation team and resuscitative endovascular balloon occlusion of the aorta. J Spec Oper Med 2017; 17(2):64–72.

74. White JM, Cannon JW, Stannard A, et al. Endovascular balloon occlusion of the aorta is superior to resuscitative thoracotomy with aortic clamping in a porcine model of hemorrhagic shock. Surgery 2011;150(3):400–9.

75. Morrison JJ, Ross JD, Houston RT, et al. Use of resuscitative endovascular balloon occlusion of the aorta in a highly lethal model of noncompressible torso hemorrhage. Shock 2014;41(2):130–7.

76. Morrison JJ, Ross JD, Rasmussen TE, et al. Resuscitative endovascular balloon occlusion of the aorta: a gap analysis of severely injured UK combat casualties. Shock 2014;41(5):388–93.

77. Stannard A, Eliason JL, Rasmussen TE. Resuscitative endovascular balloon occlusion of the aorta (REBOA) as an adjunct for hemorrhagic shock. J Trauma 2011;71(6):1869–72.

78. DuBose JJ, Scalea TM, Brenner M, et al. The AAST Prospective Aortic Occlusion for Resuscitation in Trauma and Acute Care Surgery (AORTA) Registry: data on contemporary utilization and outcomes of aortic occlusion and resuscitative balloon occlusion of the aorta (REBOA). J Trauma Acute Care Surg 2016;81(3):409–19.

79. Kuckelman JP, Barron M, Moe D, et al. Extending the golden hour for Zone 1 resuscitative endovascular balloon occlusion of the aorta. J Trauma Acute Care Surg 2018;85(2):318–26.

80. Sadek S, Lockey DJ, Lendrum RA, et al. Resuscitative endovascular balloon occlusion of the aorta (REBOA) in the pre-hospital setting: an additional resuscitation option for uncontrolled catastrophic haemorrhage. Resuscitation 2016;107: 135–8.

81. Lendrum R, Perkins Z, Chana M, et al. Pre-hospital Resuscitative Endovascular Balloon Occlusion of the Aorta (REBOA) for exsanguinating pelvic haemorrhage. Resuscitation 2019;135:6–13.

82. Lamhaut L, Qasim Z, Hutin A, et al. First description of successful use of zone 1 resuscitative endovascular balloon occlusion of the aorta in the prehospital setting. Resuscitation 2018;133:e1–2.

83. Tisherman SA, Brenner ML. Taking advanced endovascular techniques out of the hospital: ready for prime time? Resuscitation 2016;107:A3–4.

84. Northern DM, Manley JD, Lyon R, et al. Recent advances in austere combat surgery: use of aortic balloon occlusion as well as blood challenges by special operations medical forces in recent combat operations. J Trauma Acute Care Surg 2018;85(1S Suppl 2):S98–103.

85. Brenner M, Bulger EM, Perina DG, et al. Joint statement from the American College of Surgeons Committee on Trauma (ACS COT) and the American College of Emergency Physicians (ACEP) regarding the clinical use of Resuscitative Endovascular Balloon Occlusion of the Aorta (REBOA). Trauma Surg Acute Care Open 2018;3(1):e000154.

86. Allen B, Callaway D, Gibbs M, et al. Regarding the Joint Statement From the American College of Surgeons Committee on Trauma and the American College

of Emergency Physicians Regarding the Clinical Use of Resuscitative Endovascular Balloon Occlusion of the Aorta. J Emerg Med 2018;55(2):266–8.

87. de Schoutheete JC, Fourneau I, Waroquier F, et al. Three cases of resuscitative endovascular balloon occlusion of the aorta (REBOA) in austere pre-hospital environment: technical and methodological aspects. World J Emerg Surg 2018;13:54.

88. Rees P, Waller B, Buckley AM, et al. REBOA at Role 2 Afloat: resuscitative endovascular balloon occlusion of the aorta as a bridge to damage control surgery in the military maritime setting. J R Army Med Corps 2018;164(2):72–6.

The Mental Health of Disaster Responders

Giacomo Florio, PA-C[a,b,]*, Jamla Rizek Bergman, MSN, RN, CEN, CPEN, TCRN, NREMT-P[c]

KEYWORDS

- Post-traumatic stress disorder • First responders • Mental health • DMAT
- Debriefing • Suicide • Divorce

KEY POINTS

- First responders are at an increased rate of suicide.
- First responders have a higher rate of divorce.
- First responders are the key individuals during a disaster.
- A collaboration of first responders make up DMAT.

INTRODUCTION

Disasters can strike at any time or place. Some disasters are forewarned, such as hurricanes, and some are completely unexpected, such as tornadoes, earthquakes, and terror attacks.[1,2] Disaster responders mobilize for such situations sometimes with less than 24 hours' notice. Disaster responders in the case of an expected disaster stage in the areas nearby or in an easily accessible area to rapidly deploy out of. Disaster responders need to be flexible and mobilize at a moment's notice. With rapid mobilization, many natural or man-made disasters can produce an overwhelming disruption to one's social, familial, and economic wellbeing. This can create an undue amount of stress in a providers' life. This article discusses who disaster responders are, the stressors disaster responders may face, and the resources available to them.

THE DISASTER RESPONDER DEFINED

Disaster responders are usually made up of a wide array of professional and volunteer organizations with varying levels of disaster experience. Those who are involved in the disaster response vary greatly in their professions. According to Title 6 – Domestic

Disclosure Statement: Neither of us have any disclosures at this time.
[a] St. James Hospital, 411 Canisteo Street, Hornell, NY 14843, USA; [b] Emergency Department, Highland Hospital, 1000 South Avenue, Rochester, NY 14620, USA; [c] Detroit Medical Center Sinai Grace Hospital, 6071 Outer Dr. W Detroit, MI 48235, USA
* Corresponding author.
E-mail addresses: GIACOMO_FLORIO@URMC.ROCHESTER.EDU (G.F.); jamlabergman@gmail.com (J.R.B.)

Physician Assist Clin 4 (2019) 795–804
https://doi.org/10.1016/j.cpha.2019.06.007
2405-7991/19/© 2019 Elsevier Inc. All rights reserved.

Security of the United States Code, Disaster responders include the individuals and groups listed in **Table 1**.

The term emergency response providers includes federal, state, and local government and nongovernment emergency public safety, fire, law enforcement, emergency response, emergency medical and related personnel, agencies, and authorities.[3–5] Also, many NGOs, churches, and other organizations respond to a disaster. These individuals leave their families and their work behind, to be able to focus on the mission at hand. Whether that mission is a planned event such as in staging for a potential disaster, for events such as the State of the Union, or a disaster that just happened such as massive flooding, or an act of nature, disaster responders provide the care that is needed at that time with the resources that are available to them.

Many individuals play a role in disaster response. Teams may be made up of doctors, physician assistants, nurse practitioners, nurses, paramedics, and pharmacists. Pharmacists are invaluable members of a disaster team, as they can aid providers and give alternatives to medication that a provider may be used to using and let them know what is actually available in the supplied cache (medications that are available to a deployment team). The logistics team is another group within the disaster team that can help reduce a provider's stress in that team members have the know how to keep teams functioning and supplies replenished including having a plan on how to get additional supplies when the supplies run out. A profession some may be surprised to learn that is represented on a disaster team is a radiology technician, not the person who helps with the radiographs and computed tomography scans in the hospital, but the person who is familiar with radioactive material and is aware of time, distance, and shielding in the case of radioactive contamination.

Federal teams are comprised of individuals who are readily available to leave their work and lives behind to provide medical care when needed. This can be challenging for several reasons. Not only is it difficult for an individual to just leave their work and life behind and be expected to provide care to individuals who have just been hit with a disaster, but there are many emotions that go along with it. There is the potential responders to not be mentally prepared, because they are focusing on everything they must do at home or perhaps did not get a chance to since they left so rapidly.

Whether they are responding to a hurricane, flood, or other natural disaster; protecting health and saving lives in the wake of a terrorist attack or man-made disaster; providing support in the wake of a disease outbreak; or supporting a major event like the presidential inauguration, DMAT and disaster teams provide care that matters (www.phe.gov).

THE ROLE OF THE DISASTER RESPONDER

The role of the medical providers is to provide care with the resources at hand to provide the greatest good to the greatest number of people. This is not always an easy

Table 1 Disaster responders	
DMAT: Disaster Medical Assistance Team	WHO: World Health Organization
USAR: Urban Search and Rescue	American Red Cross
IMSURT: International Medical Surgical Team	MRC: Medical Reserve Corps
DEA: Drug Enforcement Agency	Logistics
NGO: Nongovernmental Organization	Wildlife and forestry
EMS: Emergency Medical Services	Engineers

task, as some of the tools that the provider may be used to having readily available at his or her daily work are not available during a disaster. There needs to be a switch in the brain of the responders to delineate their role during a disaster to not get discouraged when supplies they need are not readily available. Also, during disaster triage when providers are putting a tag on individuals: black for deceased, red for critical, yellow for moderate and green for walking wounded, providers are faced with stressors. That is, if the responders were not in a disaster zone, there would be a full hospital on hand and the ability to perform a work-up and utilize all resources. This becomes difficult, as providers must rely on physical examination skills and gut instinct, which can provide stress if providers are unsure.

During a deployment, a mix comprised of individuals from different states with different levels of experience comes together and work to care for the population in whatever tragedy is current. Not only is it a challenge working with unfamiliar teammates, but it is also hard to do with limited resources, in an unfamiliar area, with a disaster going on. Infrastructure destruction may make it more difficult for supplies to come in and patients to get transported out. Clashes of personalities, working together, stress of sleeping on floors, poor toilets, collapsed buildings, finding bodies, not enough food, supplies looted, following orders, mobilizing to different locations, and working with unknown teams are added stressors that may make the task at hand more difficult.

A BOO (base of operation), needs to get set-up so that individuals know where to come for medical care. The BOO can also be used for command purposes and as sleeping quarters for the responders. A BOO takes time to set up and build and when there is a mix of individuals, some of whom may be experts and others who may be novices, it only adds to the frustration. When there are hundreds of patients lined up, and there are people yelling, as well as no time or place to take a break or to be alone, this adds to the mental frustration. Not to mention food that one might not like to eat, and one gets so busy that one begins to suffer from dehydration and diarrhea. The pharmacy supplies limited medications, and there is a lack of resources. so walking across the street to get some Imodium for one's diarrhea is not realistic. Depending on the location in which the BOO is located, the logistics for an evacuation may be near impossible; therefore, patients are not moving or getting a higher level of care that they may need and look to the provider with longing eyes. The lack of options for them makes one feel worse.

PREDISASTER PREPAREDNESS AND STRESSORS

There are many risk factors for disaster responders, and these factors are based on time relative to the disaster. As much as one prepares for a disaster, there is always something that happens that one does not expect. It is suggested that collateral behavioral health damage in disaster responders may owe to being unfit mentally or physically prior to the disaster, as well as inadequate training, or unrealistic expectations from leadership.[6–8] Once a disaster has struck, it is too late to go back and think, "if I did this then…" Disaster responders must deal with the situation at hand as it presents itself. This goes along with mental wellbeing. As much as one can prepare for a disaster, there are so many unknowns and situations that arise that affect people in unexpected ways. This is why disaster responders prepare many things in their professional and personal life prior to responding to a disaster.

Skills

First responders train for this day in and day out by ensuring their credentials, such as basic life support (BLS), advanced cardiac life support (ACLS), and pediatric advanced life support (PALS) are up to date. Being competent, skilled providers who are active in providing patient care daily is essential. Not only is being up to date on skills important, but keeping a bag of personal items that the responder will need during a deployment is just as important.

Ready To Go

Disaster responders know from experience that they may not have the time to go home and pack. They may get their orders and be told that they need to be at the airport or central staging area within a short period of time. Responders prepare by having their uniforms and other essentials ready to go in their deployment bag. This includes a supply of any daily medication and toiletry items.

Personal

Leaving behind spouses and children can be difficult. Having the support from one's significant other will make the stress of leaving home to deploy less stressful. Not knowing whether there will be cellular service or how long it will take to get it can be scary for families who cannot reach loved ones, and the stress of them not knowing how we are or that we made it, only increases their anxieties and fears. Children are impacted by what they see on television and what they hear in school. Having the conversation with them prior to leaving puts them at ease and also gives them a sense of pride in the work that one is doing.

Financial

A deployment can be at least 2 weeks long, and not getting a paycheck from work during that time can be a financial burden, not to mention the effect it has on family left behind. Thus, it is recommended that finances be in check prior to deployment. Family members should be made aware of what accounts to use should there be an emergency at home including prioritization of bills and other expenses. Most government deployments are paid; however, it is at times approximately 50% to 75% less than their normal salary. Because the individual is getting paid, the employer does not have to pay the employee for the time that he or she deployed.

Uniformed Services Employment and Reemployment Rights Act

"The Uniformed Services Employment and Reemployment Rights Act of 1994 (USERRA) is a federal law that establishes rights and responsibilities for uniformed service members and their civilian employers".[9] Deployment orders for responders comply with USERRA, which protects them from losing their job while working a disaster. There may be some discord with the employer; however, it is crucial that the employer know upfront so that there are no "surprises" when the individual must leave. One can never predict the disaster that can occur; however, being upfront and honest is important. This also shows how dedicated one is to the profession and gives the organization a sense of pride in the work that the emergency responder is doing.

MENTAL HEALTH AND FIELD STRESSORS
Mental Health

In austere medical conditions, mental health professionals and psychiatric facilities will usually be inadequate or nonexistent. For this it is important to be able to recognize when a disaster responder is having a hard time dealing with stress. In Kenneth V. Iserson's book "Improvised Medicine," he categorizes 3 categories of crisis induced psychiatric illnesses (**Table 2**).

Table 2	
Three categories of crisis-induced psychiatric illnesses	
Adequate functioning	Most people during a crisis or disaster function at this level. They are able to cope with their feelings until they return, or things return to a normal setting.
Anxious and agitated	Distress individuals that demonstrate their crisis by loud or unmistakable crying, screaming, fainting or signs of panic, or histrionic behavior. Some may convert distress into physical signs or symptoms.
Shocked and subdued	These individuals may wander aimlessly or sit and stare. Physical signs may include confusion or disorientation.

Data from Iserson K. Improvised medicine, providing care in extreme environments. New York: McGraw Hill Education; 2020. p. 522.

Stressors

Stressors with which disaster responders can subconsciously affect the work that they are trying to do. Some stressors with which responders deal are listed in **Box 1**.

These responders are faced with the task of making life or death decisions in a split instant that can change the lives of so many, and while this holds true, providers must remember to take care of their emotional wellbeing when faced with this. Responders are prepared to face the critical incidences of their job. However, what they do not prepare for is how these incidences will affect them emotionally, after they leave the job. These responders put others first and because of their selflessness, their personal lives may pay the price. Responding to disasters can be both rewarding and challenging work. Because of this, protecting the population's health is a vital part of preserving national security and the continuity of critical national functions.

Traumatic Events

Working in a disaster can be a traumatic event for some responders. The situations are so unlike what they experience in their daily jobs. Chronic exposure to traumatic events, or even just daily stressors at work increase the likelihood that disaster

Box 1	
Disaster responders stressors	

Anxiety: The individual is on edge and may exhibit signs of uneasiness, restlessness or the inability to relax.

Depression: Weeks and months after the disaster, the responder may feel empty, lost, confused, and may suffer from the inability to communicate how they are feeling as a result of the incident.

Flashbacks: A smell, taste or sound can trigger a specific call or event that the first responder replays in their mind over and over.

Guilt: The responder may feel as though he or she did not do enough or could have done more.

Regret: The responder may feel this way if he or she was sleeping when the disaster happened and was not able to respond initially, or perhaps the individual needed to leave for his or her own mental well-being, and an adverse event happened, and they regret not being there.

Post-traumatic stress disorder (PTSD): Social pressures and lack of support can lead to lasting effects.

Substance abuse: The inability to cope with the event or compounded events may lead the individual to turn to alcohol as a way to mask his or her feelings.

responders will suffer from mental health outcomes such as depression, PTSD, chronic fatigue, increased alcohol use, potential spousal abuse, and a general poorer quality of life.[10]

Post-Traumatic Stress Disorder

Any traumatic event can cause PTSD or other stress related conditions. During a disaster, this can be caused by exposure to the dead, dying, or mutilation of bodies; chronic exposure to injured individuals; hearing the cries of the trapped or those that are in pain; or when the disaster was unexpected.

One of the core risk factors for any disaster responder is the pace of work. Disaster Responders are always on the front line facing highly stress and risky jobs. This tempo can lead to the inability to recover in between events.

Providers have their own ways of mentally preparing for a disaster; however, what works for one individual may not work for another. Having a support system is crucial to mental health wellbeing. Providers believe that there is a strong relationship between disaster responders, and it is important that they have the ability to reach out to someone who has been in the disaster with them. Some responders find it difficult to talk about what happened with their families while others feel, no one would understand.

During a disaster, social support appears to be important, particularly with having good relations with leadership and coworkers. Having supportive, approachable leaders and camaraderie among responders helps with psychological wellbeing.[11] During a disaster there is so much going on, that the effects the disaster had on the disaster responder may not be apparent until he or she is back in their normal environment. It may not hit a disaster responder until after he or she is home and back at work, all that happened on deployment. Rather than speaking to his or her family about it, the disaster responder may not want to burden loved ones, show vulnerability, or even expect that loved ones will understand.

Being able to reach out to other team members who were there may be helpful; however, this is essentially requiring the disaster responders to convince themselves that they need to talk. This may be felt as a sign of weakness and might make them feel exposed or embarrassed, so the reaching out and talking might not happen. The disaster responders then lets the feelings subconsciously get in the way, and those feelings start to affect their daily lives, unbeknownst to them. It is not uncommon for disaster responders to relate to the things they have seen and personify them.

As much as one prepares for daily jobs everyday by getting up, having a routine, and focusing on the task at hand, there are things that happen that are out of one's control. How one responds to this is important, because one needs to be able to focus on the end results and how one can get there despite the obstacles that got thrown in the way. These are just road blocks, and every disaster responder understands, that despite training, there will be a time when something comes up for which they did not train.

Burnout

The emotional stress of being deployed and addressing all the other needs mentioned previously can cause the provider to get burnout. Disaster responders always give their best, but when they begin to think that their best is not good enough or that the demands of the mission exceed their abilities, there is increased risk for burnout.

According to a study, 69% of EMS professionals have never had enough time to recover between traumatic events.[12] As a result of this, depression, stress, PTSD, and suicidal ideation have been reported. When a spouse is not in the same line of work, he or she may not understand what his or her loved one is going through at work, and this can become a challenge.

Communication issues are not uncommon, especially among disaster responders and their families. A man who sees countless domestic abuse situations may feel more strongly about the situation; however, he is also more likely to become an abuser himself. This is because he has no outlet to express his feelings. He feels as though no one understands and thus takes out his aggression on those who are closest to him.

The Ruderman Foundation studied suicide among disaster responders and found that firefighters and police officers are 20% more likely to commit suicide than anyone else.[13–16]

SOLUTIONS

One cannot fix anything unless one first acknowledges that this is an issue with which disaster responders are faced. Support is important, not only at home, but in the workplace as well. Nonverbal and verbal queues are what people pick up, on and they need to not be afraid to speak up and reach out and express their concern over one's well-being. This cannot be one-sided. The responder must feel comfortable talking about how he or she is feeling and understanding that expressing his or her emotions does not make them weak or less of a person. First responders may hide behind a strong exterior, when behind it, they are crumbling. Recognizing a change in one's loved one and getting him or her help even when he or she says he or she is fine and does not need help can prevent a tragedy later on.

Debriefing

Disaster and emergency personnel are not exempt from the devastating impact of tragic events on their emotions, health, careers, family, or lives. In fact, they may be more seriously affected because of the ability to suppress their reactions to maintain their ability to function in times of stress and may fear their emotions and fear debilitation. Therefore, debriefing is a way most agencies have helped reduce the mental baggage brought back from a disaster or crisis. This is a way for one to let out his or her feelings and fears.

Although there are some individuals who take debriefing lightly, others engage in the conversation and open up about how the situation made them feel and how they are coping with what they saw during the disaster. Talking about feelings is not an easy thing to do, especially when one consider how the media identify the majority of disaster responders as men. There is a fear that their peers will treat first responders differently and the stigma of not being able to handle the job or being weak. However, by opening up and discussing the event and how it makes them feel and how it is affecting them, it may give someone else the opportunity to open up also, perhaps someone who was internally struggling and was afraid to reach out for help. It is important that agencies develop a clear line of communication and develop mental health and resilience training and promote counseling following stressful situations.

It is important to note that a debriefing is not an opportunity for someone to place blame on another person, nor is it the time to talk about how things could have or should gave gone, but rather to reflect on the event or situation after it has happened and to discuss how what happened affects first responders. There is an opportunity to provide feedback as to opportunities for improvement. This is important, because from this one can learn ways to better adapt to situations in future deployments.

Those who came to help others in their time of need were thought to be trained not to react to human carnage and destruction or to the pain of the survivors. They were considered exempt from the psychological complications that result from disasters. In reality, this is not true. These events impact their health, careers, family, and their lives. Health responders are more seriously affected, because disaster responders are in the habit of suppressing their reactions and emotions in order to maintain the ability to function during any crisis and later because they might fear debilitation from their own emotions within their own personal lives.

In terms of DMAT, teammates have a routine of debriefing daily before leaving the area where working and before heading back to the sleeping barracks. The goal of this is to be able to discuss things that happened during the shift, plan for the next day, and also highlight some of the things that went well or could have gone better. It is also important to show appreciation for the members of the team for the things that they have done.

RESOURCES

If you or someone you know is having a hard time coping with a disaster, do not be afraid to reach out. Talk to someone. You are not alone. One should not make the mistake of taking care of everyone else but forgetting to take care of oneself. Providers need to be vigilant in their awareness of changes in behavior, suicidal comments, or peers being withdrawn. Mental health providers are available. Providers need to not be afraid to reach out. There are many campaigns that support disaster responders, and social media platforms have become a great outlet for responders to connect with one another.

The CODE Green Campaign provides awareness and education on PTSD in disaster responders. The Code Green Campaign is raising awareness on mental health issues that affect disaster responders, and also providing education to those who think that they should just deal with it or it is part of the job. However, public health workers can experience a broad range of health and mental health consequences because of work-related exposures to natural or human-caused disasters.[17]

The National Suicide Prevention Lifeline is a 24/7/365 free phone call that provides confidential support for anyone, not just disaster responders. This is a confidential call.

The Disaster Responders Support Network (DRSN) not only has a retreat for disaster responders, but also for their spouses, which is crucial to healing after a traumatic incident. The great thing about this organization is that it is run by volunteers. The DRSN discusses secondary traumatization, which is when the individual listening to the story, such as the spouse of the responder, is affected by his or her firsthand experiences. Secondary traumatization is not discussed so openly; however, it can also lead to communication barriers.

Backing the Badge is an organization that shows support for law enforcement agencies and highlights the work that they do along with the dangers that go along with it. This organization has not branched in all the states, but the ones in which they have a presence have incredibly active social media pages that include pictures, community events, and words of support. By highlighting all of this, law enforcement officers have the ability to see the good that they do and cope with the traumatic events with which they have to deal on a daily basis.

Share the Load program highlights the mental health issues in disaster responders, specifically firefighters. One of the concerns is how physically capable these men and women are, but they may not be able to mentally cope with what goes on at work every day. The alarm goes off, and they are on that fire truck, sometimes not even taking a moment's rest between calls and still maintaining their professionalism and dedication to the community they serve.

Only a few of the available organizations that are out there in support of and for disaster responders are mentioned here, but the key factor is recognizing the abnormal or withdrawn behavior and being able to feel comfortable asking for or reaching out for help. There is no shame in that.

When one factors in all the issues that go on in the lives of the disaster responders every day and then one takes them away from that environment to deploy to a disaster with individuals from different states and skill levels with limited resources, it is not only mentally challenging, but exhausting also. First responders must be able to do the work for which they trained, and hey cannot do that without support at home from their families, coworkers, and employers.

SUMMARY

Being a first responder emits a sense of pride in the work that is done to provide care to individuals that are unable to care for themselves. Being able to provide this service is gratifying and fulfilling. However, there is more to it than just being there when needed. Responding to disasters plays a toll on one's emotions and in one's daily lives. Daily career work may be affected, because providers are gone for weeks at a time. Personal lives also may be affected when loved ones do not understand why one would want to leave them and work during a disaster that is stressful and hard work. Difficult emotions can get the best of providers when working with individuals who have different personalities and with whom one is not accustomed to working alongside. Disaster responders can tire easily and feel burned out because of the situation, and sad because they wish we could do more for those that were affected. The money made does not pay the bills and can create financial stress. Sleep may be affected, as one may be sleeping in crowded spaces, during odd hours, and in sleeping bags.

With that being said, there is something so gratifying about being able to respond to a disaster that disaster responders take all those facts and prepare for the effects it will have and mentally put emotions in check and move on. Disaster responders understand that it is not easy, but still do it out of passion. The relationships made on deployments with other responders are lasting ones. Although disaster responders may not speak to each other on a daily basis, they will forever have a shared experience that others at home may not understand.

REFERENCES

1. Abbot C, Barber E, Burke B, et al. What's killing our medics? 2015. Available at: http://www.revivingresponders.com/originalpaper. Accessed February 7, 2019.
2. Benedek DM, Fullerton C, Ursano RJ. Disaster responders: mental health consequences of natural and human-made disasters for public safety workers. Annu Rev Public Health 2007. https://doi.org/10.1146/annurev.pubhealth.28.021406. 144037.
3. Domestic Security, 6 U.S.C. 101. Available at: https://www.gpo.gov/fdsys/pkg/USCODE-2010-title6/pdf/USCODE-2010-title6-chap1.pdf. Accessed February 20, 2019.
4. Available at: http://codegreencampaign.org/. Accessed February 20, 2019.
5. Available at: https://www.firerescue1.com/fire-rehab/articles/2181154-Firefighter-divorce-3-important-facts/. Accessed February 20, 2019.
6. Mitchell JT. Collateral damage in disaster workers. Int J Emerg Ment Health 2011; 13(2):121–5.
7. Available at: http://www.frsn.org/. Accessed April 6, 2019.

8. Available at: https://www.nvfc.org/programs/share-the-load-program/. Accessed April 6, 2019.

9. Available at: https://www.esgr.mil/USERRA/What-is-USERRA. Accessed April 6, 2019.

10. Arble et al., 2017.

11. Brooks SK, Dunn R, Amlot R, et al. Social and occupational factors associated with psychological distress and disorder among disaster responders. A systematic review. BMC Psychol 2016;4:18.

12. Bentley MA, Crawford JM, Watkins JR, et al. An assessment of depression, anxiety, and stress among nationally certified EMS professionals. Prehosp Emerg Care 2013;17(3):330–8.

13. Available at: https://www.lawenforcementtoday.com/suicide-rates-Disaster-responders-20-percent-higher-public/. Accessed May 29, 2019.

14. Available at: https://www.phe.gov/preparedness/responders/ndms/ndms-teams/pages/dmat.aspx. Accessed May 29, 2019.

15. Iserson K. Improvised medicine, providing care in extreme environments 2012. Mcgraw Hill Eduction; 2011. p. 522.

16. Marmar CR, McCaslin SE, Metzler TJ, et al. Predictors of posttraumatic stress in police and other Disaster responders. Ann N Y Acad Sci 2006;1071:1–18. Available at: https://search-ebscohost-com.contentproxy.phoenix.edu/login.aspx?direct=true&db=mdc&AN=16891557&site=ehost-live&scope=site.

17. Benedek, et al. First responders: Mental health consequences of natural and Human made disasters for Public health and Public safety workers. Annual Review of Public Health 2007;28:55–68.

Moving?

Make sure your subscription moves with you!

To notify us of your new address, find your **Clinics Account Number** (located on your mailing label above your name), and contact customer service at:

Email: **journalscustomerservice-usa@elsevier.com**

800-654-2452 (subscribers in the U.S. & Canada)
314-447-8871 (subscribers outside of the U.S. & Canada)

Fax number: 314-447-8029

Elsevier Health Sciences Division
Subscription Customer Service
3251 Riverport Lane
Maryland Heights, MO 63043

*To ensure uninterrupted delivery of your subscription, please notify us at least 4 weeks in advance of move.